THE RESEARCH JOURNEY

The Research Journey
Introduction to Inquiry

Sharon F. Rallis
Gretchen B. Rossman

Foreword by
Thomas A. Schwandt

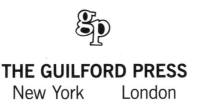

THE GUILFORD PRESS
New York   London

© 2012 The Guilford Press
A Division of Guilford Publications, Inc.
72 Spring Street, New York, NY 10012
www.guilford.com

Printed in the United States of America

This book is printed on acid-free paper.

Last digit is print number: 9   8   7   6   5   4   3   2   1

Library of Congress Cataloging-in-Publication Data

Rallis, Sharon F.
   The research journey : introduction to inquiry / Sharon F. Rallis, Gretchen B.
Rossman.
      p.   cm.
   Includes bibliographical references and index.
   ISBN 978-1-4625-0512-8 (pbk.)—ISBN 978-1-4625-0514-2 (hardcover)
   1. Dissertations, Academic.   2. Research—Methodology—Study and
teaching (Graduate).   I. Rossman, Gretchen B..   II. Title.
   LB2369.R35 2012
   808.02—dc23

                                                              2011049299

To all the road trips we have taken
and to those in our dreams

Foreword

In the professional practice fields of social work, nursing, education, and so forth—just as in the disciplines—inquiring minds want to know answers to basic questions about individual and collective behavior: What is happening here? Why did it happen? How did it happen? What does it mean? What are the effects of its having happened? Teaching and learning how to pose meaningful questions of this kind and how to investigate them in systematic, ethically responsible, empirically defensible, and practically useful ways are demanding tasks. Multiple challenges to developing "inquiry-minded graduate students" present themselves in such an undertaking.

An early challenge arises in picturing what learning to be inquiry minded entails. Numerous textbooks present in various ways the toolbox of methods and procedures for social-behavioral inquirers who seek to collect and analyze both quantitative and qualitative data to answer important empirical questions in their fields. One can easily get the impression from such books that the process of learning to be an inquirer is a matter of following a "how-to" prescription. Learning the tools of the trade is indispensible to being a good inquirer. However, the *process* of becoming "inquiry minded" is, as Rallis and Rossman emphasize, a journey. The metaphor of a journey signifies development over time. Moreover, a journey can be a trek, an undertaking on a difficult and not necessarily straightforward path from Point *A* to Point *B*. When on a journey, one needs to be capable of dealing with detours and delays; perhaps some bad advice; perhaps some backtracking; and often indecision about the best next move. To be sure, the journey has a "destination," as the authors put it—the process of inquiry "ends" with some kind of product. Yet, to my way of thinking, such destinations are merely temporary stopping points. The journey to becoming—and sustaining the ability and dispositions to be—inquiry minded is never really finished.

The journey requires a number of capacities. Acquiring and enhancing those capacities constitute yet another set of challenges to becoming inquiry minded. The abilities and aptitudes that make up being inquiry minded are at least threefold. First, there is the challenge of learning the language of the practice. Researchers must become adept at working with the core epistemological ideas of responsible, systematic, empirical inquiry—notions such as explanation, objectivity, subjectivity, generalization, representation, theory, evidence, justification, and warranting—as well as the more specialized vocabulary of terms such as interpretivism, constructionism, hermeneutics, standpoint, critical realism, and critical theory that influence the framing of a study's questions and theoretical perspective. Second, there is the necessity of learning that inquiry practice demands both technical and craftsman-like skills. To engage in systematic, disciplined inquiry—that is, an investigation that is well ordered, organized, methodical, and well argued—one must become expert in using some of the tools of the trade. Here, methods books are most helpful in providing advice on the design of experiments, the requirements of a good interview, the design of a good survey, the means of analyzing narrative or quantitative data, and so forth.

What these books cannot provide, however, is instruction in the capacity for practical wisdom. And this presents yet another challenge. Such wisdom is all about learning how to exercise good judgment absent any procedural rules in the many decision situations one faces as an inquirer. For example: How do I know whether I have sufficiently searched for evidence to disprove my hypotheses (the search for disconfirming evidence or negative cases)? How do I know which alternative explanations for a causal relationship that I have postulated are plausible? How many people should I interview? How extensive should my field notes be? How should I handle a breach of confidentiality? How do I assess the risks to participants involved in my field study? In the field of nursing, Patricia Benner and colleagues have identified "clinical reasoning" as a form of practical wisdom. It involves reflective, critical thinking coupled with the ability to reason in situ—to "size up" the situation as it presents itself here in this set of circumstances, at this time and place, with these particular contextual dimensions—along with an ability to identify patterns. The capacity for good judgment is something acquired through experience, through the study of cases of similar decision-making situations, through conversation with others further along in their journey, and through thoughtful conversations with peers who are making the journey to be inquiry minded.

A final challenge, intimately related to acquiring aptitudes and abilities, is cultivating intellectual habits, values, and dispositions that are the mark of scientific integrity in an inquiry-minded person. These include a commitment to fallibilism, taking seriously the notion that one can be wrong about one's beliefs or position and being open to new evidence and arguments; skepticism, the continual scrutiny of one's procedures and methods for errors as well as the search for evidence that disconfirms one's claims, assertions, or hypotheses: honesty, curiosity, objectivity, and the willingness and ability to explore suppositions and beliefs that lie behind one's research interests and agenda.

The great pragmatist philosopher Charles Sanders Peirce provided some practical advice for guiding the reasoning process that makes up becoming inquiry minded: "Upon this first, and in one sense this sole, rule of reason, that in order to learn you must desire to learn, and in so desiring not be satisfied with what you already incline to think, there follows one corollary which itself deserves to be inscribed upon every wall of the city of philosophy: Do not block the road of inquiry" (1898/1992). *The Research Journey: Introduction to Inquiry* is a text that embodies that advice and provides a reliable guide to becoming inquiry minded.

THOMAS A. SCHWANDT, PhD
University of Illinois at Urbana–Champaign

Preface

This book is a product of our several decades of teaching about research, conducting research ourselves, and advising graduate students who conducted research and of our reflections (meaning both thought and action) on the teaching and on the conduct of research. We are methodologists—we care about what is behind the methods chosen to inform questions. We are also practitioners—we do what we teach about. Most important, the book is a product of our years of collaboration—teaching and researching.

For the past 7 years, we have co-taught a course that introduces the concepts and processes of inquiry to graduate students in the social sciences and professional schools. This course had its roots in the Inquiry for Practitioners course Sharon Rallis developed and taught in the 1990s at Vanderbilt University. While the course was offered through the Peabody College of Education and Human Development, students enrolled from public policy, divinity, law, nursing, public health, and other disciplines. Because most of the students came from either the social sciences or professional schools, the purpose of the course was to make inquiry relevant and practical to people who work in fields that can be informed by research; Rallis hoped they would become capable and critical consumers and researchers. The goal was to ground practice in theory. Meanwhile, Gretchen Rossman was teaching the same types of students—those from both social science disciplines and professional schools—so her research courses also emphasized the value of informing practice through research.

Over the years of various collaborations—writing books, conducting research, coteaching, giving presentations—a new version of Inquiry has emerged. At the University of Massachusetts Amherst in the School of Education, the course has now become a required introductory inquiry course for doctoral students in several specializations. The course focuses on questions foundational to fostering inquiry mindedness in graduate students:

- What is knowledge?
- How is it produced?
- Who uses it and how?

We have found that the course—Introduction to Inquiry—serves to socialize graduate students into the world of scholars who are committed to conducting research that will contribute to human well-being. The course also serves to familiarize graduate students with the discourses, norms, and practices of academia and the research enterprise.

This book has developed from our teaching practice. Thus, our purpose is to share the course experience with you, to the extent that pedagogy in practice can be translated into a book. Therefore, we try to explicate—that is, make transparent—our pedagogy. Our audience is students and the faculty who teach them. We hope that the faculty are committed to their own learning as well as that of their students.

The book is structured to follow a teaching sequence; in fact, it maps neatly onto our syllabus for the course (changed, updated, and revised each year, of course). Each chapter begins with a series of critical questions that we hope will guide reading and prompt further questions for discussion. These questions are followed by a dialogue among five graduate students whose journeys into inquiry are just beginning. While the metaphor of journey is overused, we still find it generative to capture the notion of *inquiry as journey*. These students are modeled after very real graduate students whom we have taught. Their challenges and joys are embedded in these dialogues as well as throughout the chapters. We also draw on other examples from our students over the years in several places. The chapters end with learning activities that we have used over the years and refined, based on student feedback and our own critical reflections on how well they worked. Further readings are suggested.

Chapter 1—"Inquiry as Learning: Beginning the Journey"—presents our central argument that inquiry is all about learning and that the researcher is a learner. Chapter 2—"Ways of Knowing: Finding a Compass"—presents questions about epistemology and ontology (in ways that are grounded, we hope) to invite students to consider what some of their basic assumptions are about knowing, knowledge, and the social world. Chapter 3—"The Cycle of Inquiry: More Than One Way to Get There"—describes models of inquiry and learning that reinforce the notion that there are multiple ways to know and understand. "Being an Ethical Inquirer: Staying Alert on the Road"—Chapter 4—argues that the inquirer should be a moral practitioner whose sensibilities recognize the need to honor participants as well as meet standards for ethical practice. In this chapter, we address university-based requirements for protection of human subjects. Chapter 5—"Constructing Conceptual Frameworks: Building the Route"—takes students through the complex, exciting, confusing—and essential—processes of connecting their personal research interests with larger, historical, ongoing discourses that are relevant for their work. Students learn how to build their arguments, support them with sufficient evidence, and articulate their reasoning. "Designing the Inquiry Project: Finding 'True North'"—Chapter 6—offers several options for designing a study; it shows how designs should emerge from the conceptual framework. Chapter 7—"Things to Consider in Writing: Staying in the Right Lane"—provides detailed tips and hints about writing introductions, avoiding plagiarism, and using appropriate citation formats. Finally, Chapter 8—"Knowledge Use: Arriving at Your Destination"—considers the often-unanswered questions: What happens with what I've learned? How can it be used? Who else might care? This chapter closes the loop by revisiting the conceptual framework as the heart of any inquiry project.

We would like to acknowledge the doctoral students in our Introduction to Inquiry course over the past 3 years. Those in the 2009 cohort wrote the Prologue; the 2010 group provided critical feedback on three chapters; and the 2011 group offered not only insights and suggestions but also line edits. Our appreciation to each group. The 2009 class included Mika Abdullaeva, Gerardo Blanco Ramirez, Cheryl Brooks, Jackie Brousseau-Periera, Chris Canning-Wilson, Erica Cole, Ellie Cruz, Jeff Darling, Daniel De La Torre, Mindy Eichhorn, Sabrina Forbes, Letha Gayle-Brissett, Mohammad Javad, Martin McEvoy, Tara Pepis, Konda Chavva Reddy, Dawn Rendell, and Sara Sandstrom. The 2010 group comprised Yetunde Ajao, Sandra Andrew, Theresa Bianchi, Diana Bonneville, Michael Buoniconti, Koni Denham, Maura Devlin, Kevin Fleming, Noga Flory, Yang Gyeltshen, Emily Perlow, Tony Randall, Yedalis Ruiz, Karla Sarr, Rolf Straubhaar, Chris Tranberg, and David Vacchi. The 2011 group included Tara Brandt, Javier Campos,

Patrick Connelly, Helen-Ann Ireland, Mike de Jesus, Salma Khan, Naeem Khawaja, Alicia Remaly, Colleen Smith, and Julie Spencer-Robinson.

We also want to acknowledge the contributions of our graduate assistants over the years: Diane Murphy, Aaron Kuntz, Ian Martin, and Idene Rodriguez Martin. We are grateful for the helpful comments of the manuscript's reviewers: Sande Milton, Florida State University; Eleni Elder, Florida Atlantic University; and Arlene Andrews, University of South Carolina. Finally, this book would not have come to fruition without the gentle nudges of C. Deborah Laughton, our editor of many years. She hung in with us as we took our time with revisions. Thank you, C. Deb.

SHARON F. RALLIS, Jamestown, RI
GRETCHEN B. ROSSMAN, Amherst, MA

Contents

3 The Cycle of Inquiry: More Than One Way to Get There   39

4 Being an Ethical Inquirer: Staying Alert on the Road   57

5 Constructing Conceptual Frameworks: Building the Route   85

6 Designing the Inquiry Project: Finding "True North"   111

7 Things to Consider in Writing: Staying in the Right Lane   139

Prologue

GREETINGS TO BEGINNING INQUIRERS[1]:

As survivors of the first year in graduate study, we second-year students want to welcome you as you begin your first "real" graduate-level course. This course is unique because it challenges what you currently think you know. As you might expect, this is not always an easy task.

We discovered that graduate study is a journey—we covered ground—moving forward and also back; we faced obstacles and challenges; and we learned and grew. We discovered that it is different from many of our earlier experiences because we were asked to take on a new role, one where we, rather than others, interpret meaning. Because interpreting meaning is not easy, we thought we would pass along some advice—things that we've learned as part of the process. Ready? Here goes:

- What we know and how we know it are more complicated than you ever thought.
- Pace yourself—this class can demand a lot of time and effort thinking, reading, rethinking, writing, and rewriting. You'll need to give your thoughts time to "marinate" before you can write.
- Be open to others' ideas and feedback. This may help generate new

---

[1]These comments and suggestions were written by students in our *Introduction to Inquiry* course, fall 2009.

1

ideas or new ways of thinking about the topic, fine-tune existing ideas, and see other perspectives.

- Develop comfort with ambiguity. All of us are grappling with the topic and learning how to draft a proposal. At times, it feels like groping in the dark. Be assured that the professors are aware of this. Learn to become comfortable with ambiguity. This is a critical skill that will stand you in good stead as you progress along in your research!

- At times this class may feel very heady and theoretical; be okay with the discomfort this causes. You will likely encounter words, terms, and concepts that you have not heard before. Don't be shy about asking for definitions and explanations if you don't feel satisfied with your understanding.

- Use this class as an opportunity to get feedback and to see the world in new ways: complete assignments even when they feel like they don't make sense; don't be discouraged when the feedback you receive is negative or critical, and don't be afraid to ask for more.

- Feel free to experiment with creativity. There is no one right way; you will develop your style for inquiry. You can be more creative with your project than you may think.

- What you get from this course depends on your efforts and attitude—approaching inquiry (and the course) with a positive attitude helps.

- *You* are responsible for your own learning, so invest in the process to become an independent thinker. Allow yourself to experiment, feel discomfort, make mistakes, and be patient with the different stages of learning.

Finally, you will hear yourself asking again and again: What do I know, and how do I know it? Go ahead and question and doubt everything *except* your ability to succeed in this class. At times, you may feel overwhelmed, but you will finish—and will be pleased with the product. Learning to use the inquiry process will help you successfully move through the journey of graduate study—and to generate knowledge yourself.

Good luck—and have fun!

CHAPTER 1

Inquiry as Learning
Beginning the Journey

✳ *Critical Questions to Guide Your Reading*

⤳ *What is my role as an inquirer? (remembering)*

⤳ *What does it mean to generate knowledge? (understanding)*

⤳ *How does my interest in a topic help shape what I want to learn? (applying)*

⤳ *How do the experiences of scientists relate to my work? (applying)*

⤳ *Does inquiry take multiple forms? (analyzing)*

⤳ *What understanding of inquiry seems to best suit my project? (evaluating)*

Dialogue 1. What *Is* Inquiry?

Four students in the university's professional schools (business, education, public health, and public policy) and one in the social sciences are beginning their graduate study. As first-year students, they are enrolled in a cross-discipline seminar that aims to socialize them into academia. After their first *Introduction to Inquiry* class, they are gathering up their belongings before leaving the classroom. Professor Bettara has just left, and they strike up a conversation.

RAUL: Hey, this course sounds like just what I need . . . formal permission to question everything. And I'm always looking for new ways to see the world. By the way, I'm in the business school.

KEVIN: No way! What's all this about how do we know what we know? Don't I either know something or not? I'm a school principal, so I don't have time to play around. I need answers.

MARTINA: I want answers too, but I realize that they are not just hanging from trees for me to pick. In my field, public health, we have plenty of problems and plenty of solutions, but they don't often match. I come from a small village in Africa so I've seen the experts bring solutions by the dozens. And most don't work because they were designed for other places with different ways of seeing the world. Isn't that what Bettara said the course is about? Different ways of knowing? And how to raise questions that open up possibilities? That works for me.

SAMIRA: Me too. I like that idea about taking on Truth, that truth is related to cultural norms and socialization. I've been working in poor communities, and the people there would sure say that their truths weren't the same as people's in the suburbs. I'm in public policy, but I'm especially interested in social justice, so I'm hoping the readings will help me question policies effectively.

KEVIN: Did you look at that reading list? Way too much!

REILLY: Yes, well, I already know a lot from my master's degree in political science. I'm starting this doctorate in political science so I can hone my research skills.

RAUL: I hate to be difficult, but I have to ask what you mean when you say you already know a lot. I'd guess that Bettara would question whether you're sure you know a lot from getting a degree.

KEVIN: All I know is that everything sounds complex and confusing. How do we do inquiry? Are there steps to follow? I'm going to count on you folks to help me through.

SAMIRA: Aha! See? We are already asking questions. And so our inquiry begins.

This introductory dialogue among student learners invites you to begin to engage with the key questions and purposes of this book. We introduce each chapter with a short dialogue among people like you who are setting out to do an inquiry project and are baffled and excited, all at the same time. We introduce these students (whose characteristics and interests, we note, are drawn from real students who have taken our classes) more fully in Chapter 2.

INTRODUCTION

The opening dialogue and the Prologue letter from our former students should evoke several questions that will be central to your journey as graduate students: What is knowledge? How do we know that we know something? What does it mean to "produce knowledge"? And, what is inquiry? To begin to engage with these questions, we turn to 20th-century educational philosopher Israel Scheffler, who problematizes the concept "knowledge," as we do throughout this book. Troubling your understanding of "knowledge" is central to our purposes because if knowledge is seen as problematic—that is, complicated, full of twists and turns—space opens up to talk explicitly about inquiry.

Scheffler (1965) puts forward three claims, arguing that in order to know something the following conditions must be met:

1. I believe it is true;
2. I have evidence that it is true; and
3. It is true.

At first glance, the first two criteria seem relatively straightforward: I believe something and I have evidence to support that belief. For example, I believe that the weather is hot, and I have looked at the thermometer, which indicates a temperature of 90° Fahrenheit. I'm also sweating. However, the third criterion complicates matters: If I believe the weather is hot and I have evidence, is it not, therefore, "true" that it is hot? Surely, it would be oxymoronic to say that I know something that I also know to be false. However, the truth condition implies that I am not mistaken in my commitment to the first two conditions. But who is to judge if I am mistaken in my belief that it is hot? Perhaps it depends on the credibility of the evidence that I put forward. If sweat and a reading on the thermometer convince me that it is hot, then one could argue that I "know" it is hot. However, persons from a different climate might regard 90° Fahrenheit as moderate; to them, the evidence is not convincing of "hotness." They would not say that a claim of hotness meets the truth condition.

Suddenly, knowledge claims become problematic. With matters about the physical environment, evidence may be more easily agreed to; with matters of the social world and human actions, however, evidence and claims of knowledge are essentially contested. We stand not on *terra firma* but on *terra mobila*. Other philosophers (see especially Williams, 2001) have unpacked this tricky criterion—the claim that something is true—suggesting that knowing is a dynamic process with self-corrective and recursive elements; that is, counterbeliefs or counterevidence emerges and opens up the possibility of altering what we claim we know and, thus, determinations of truth.

But what counts as evidence? Do beliefs count as evidence? If so, to whom? And under what conditions? Scheffler's criteria, while apparently elegant and simple, upon close inspection provoke us to consider that knowing involves both fact—some sort of tangible evidence perhaps—and value—who is assessing that evidence. And central to knowing, and making claims about what we know, is this process that we call inquiry. Inquiry may confirm what we already "know" (it's hot because I'm sweating) or it may result in a new way of seeing the world, a discovery (I'm hot but my colleague from India is not; that's a fascinating notion).

> How do we know *what* we know? How do we know *that* we know?

This chapter explores the process of *inquiry*, a natural human and social endeavor that confirms or elaborates existing knowledge and can generate new knowledge. The obvious question that follows is, What is knowledge? Therefore, we consider definitions of knowledge, including the corollary concept *learning*. We consider who the learner is and how the learner's biography, values, and passions shape the inquiry and the resulting knowledge, and we relate inquiry to research and scientific discovery, as well as to babies in cribs.

The inquiry process problematizes knowledge because it highlights that what we take as knowledge may not be what it seems. Thus, the inquiry process may result in confirming existing knowledge, elaborating that knowledge, or generating new knowledge. Whatever the result, we think differently about what we thought we knew or what we claimed we thought we knew. The inquiry process invites us to ask the questions: *What* do we know about our world? *How* do we know what we know? Even more basic, how do we know *that* we know? These questions address Scheffler's first two criteria for knowing and lead into discussions about *ontology* (what we take as reality) and *epistemology* (how we know this reality). Inquiry also engages with Scheffler's third query: Given how I know what I know, can I call this knowledge true? As we explore ontology and epistemology, we also examine additional complex terms like *ideology, paradigm, conceptualization and reconceptualization, theory,* and *standpoint.* Each of these terms represents concepts at the heart of the inquiry process, ones we revisit throughout the book. To simplify, however, the practice of inquiry is learning.

The goal of this text is to engage you, the student, in learning, through readings and activities that foster a critical questioning—an inquiry—of your own knowledge and encourage you to see that all knowledge is limited, partial, and socially and historically situated, and emerges from a complex mix of socialization and experience. Most important, as you assume your emergent role as participant in the research community, we challenge you to discover, articulate, and use your own ways of knowing to inquire and generate knowledge. This book can be your guide.

Taking on this role is challenging, as many students come to graduate school with the notion that there is one *Truth* or a generally accepted knowledge that exists about a topic or issue or problem of practice that they are interested in. We have found that students from all over the world, including the United States, may hold this epistemological assumption about the nature of truth as a result of socialization or cultural norms. In fact, one powerful form of socialization that commonly encourages the acceptance of the one right answer is traditional schooling, where students are seen as vessels to be filled with extant knowledge. Similarly, students may hail from cultural groups where the prevailing epistemology does not admit for other than the Word (whether from an authority figure, a religious text, or another). Thus, we have seen that students sometimes struggle with alternative worldviews, seeking confirmation of their existing beliefs; discovery and exploration are daunting.

What is truth?

Our perspective is different; we believe knowledge is both individually and socially constructed from among many possible truths. We see knowledge as dynamic, not definitive, ever growing and changing. Knowledge is both a product of social interaction and a factor contributing to social change (Berger & Luckmann, 1967). If any inquiry process is to have merit, we must allow for possible differing perspectives or "findings" that may alter our initial beliefs or understandings or at least more fully explain where our understandings and beliefs come from. Thus, we present inquiry as dynamic and ultimately socially constructed.

While we recognize many processes that generate knowledge, we are academics, so we discuss knowledge production through systematic inquiry, a formalized process of questions, designs, and methods to conduct genera-tive research. Our value stance is that such research should contribute to growth and human well-being. Because our own backgrounds are in edu-cation, many of our examples focus on U.S. PreK–12 public schools, non-formal education settings, higher education, and international development education. Aware that many readers may come from other fields, we craft our examples to be relevant to noneducators, including those from health, government, and other social service areas. We explore the intersection of theory and practice, with emphasis on the epistemological assumptions and design of thoughtful, ethical inquiry.

Our purpose in this text is to foster inquiry-minded graduate stu-dents—those who can recognize an anomaly or problem or curiosity; frame it as a question, hypothesis, or argument; design and conduct a systematic process to inform the question, test the hypothesis, or investigate the argu-ment; and interpret what is found or learned for an appropriate audience. As an inquiry-minded graduate student, you will uncover assumptions and experiences that you bring to research and become sensitive to the variety of ways the social world can be viewed and interpreted. You will consider consequences of a given worldview and its attending actions. You will inter-rogate the assumptions underlying the questions or arguments and be open to alternative views and to modifying your views and your actions. Inquiry-minded graduate students exemplify what science has called modern man: *Homo sapiens sapiens*, that is, one who knows that he knows. The term *Homo sapiens* derives from the Latin verb *sapere*, to know. This book, and the process of systematic inquiry that you will engage in, is part of becoming explicitly sapient, or knowing.

Graduate students quickly learn that one requirement for obtaining their degree is conducting some original research. The word *research* is thus emblematic of graduate study. Some students approach their studies with an idea of what they want to learn; others may even have a specific research question in mind. Some even may come knowing what they want to find and expect their research to prove what they already know. More often, however, students arrive in graduate school with a broad area of interest and perhaps a vague understanding of what is meant by "research." Some even come merely for the credentialing of an advanced degree and so do not bring a research interest. A boundary note: This book is not about research per se or about research methods; it is about inquiry, a much more encompassing and, we believe, more important term—more encompassing and more important because, as the policy of the Council of Graduate Schools in the United States (1977) declares, graduate programs are meant to prepare a student for a lifetime of intellectual inquiry that manifests itself in scholarship and research. But, you ask: What exactly *is* inquiry?

WHAT IS INQUIRY?

First and foremost, inquiry is a natural process that you, because you are a thinking being, have engaged in since you were born. You are curious about what you see, hear, touch, taste, and smell, so you question your world. You gather data (the building blocks of information) through these senses, you find patterns in them, and ultimately you make meaning of what your senses bring you. You make meaning of the world; that is, through a "sense-making process" (Weick, 1995), you construct much of your way of knowing the natural and human-designed worlds. Usually, you are not aware of the process, but as your questions become more complex and sophisticated, you discover or create and use explicit processes for the inquiry. Ultimately, you move from using only your innate sense making to explicitly employing tools of systematic inquiry. Thus, inquiry implies involvement in "a conscious process of curiosity that guides planned, strategic exploration and investigation" (Brunk-Chavez & Foster, 2010b, p. 3). Inquiry includes elements of science (planning, deliberation, systematizing) and of art (curiosity, imagination, emotion).

We mentioned babies in cribs. Consider the popular book *The Scientist in the Crib* (Gopnik, Meltzoff, & Kuhl, 2001), in which the authors summarize recent research on very young babies and children and how they learn about their worlds. The authors claim that "babies formulate hypotheses, conduct experiments, reach conclusions, and revise what they know in light of new evidence—just like scientists" (Pycha, n.d.). The authors also describe

> Babies in cribs are scientists.

the incredible joy that the baby scientists experience in their work because they discover and create. As we discuss in Chapter 3, babies, graduate students, managers, scholars, and teachers all move through an inquiry cycle as they learn.

Inquiry, then, critiques, confirms, or creates knowledge; in short, you learn. Essentially, because learning can be defined as the process by which you create knowledge, inquiry *is* learning. Learning and knowledge, however, are dynamic and tentative, not definitive and providing the right answer. Learning seeks Knowledge instead of Truth. Usually, the more you know, the more you know exists out there to learn, the more you raise questions about what is known. Similarly, knowledge is more than the production of facts; the facts or data come together into patterns or images that inform issues and problems, which are then interpreted through your—the learner's—lenses. *You* make sense of these patterns.

Learning leads to deeper understanding because you gather and combine data (images, words, numbers, impressions) into information and then use the information to turn it into knowledge. Using the information is critical to knowledge production. The relationship among data/facts, information, and knowledge, although not completely linear, might best be illustrated through the following progression (see Figure 1.1):

data – info – knowledge – Power

- *Data* analyzed and synthesized become →

- *Information* interpreted and used becomes →

- *Knowledge*.

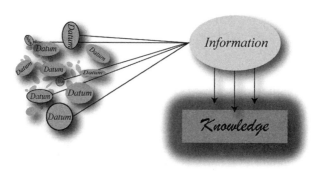

FIGURE 1.1. Data, information, knowledge.

THE LEARNER AS KNOWLEDGE GENERATOR

Emphasis on inquiry as learning shifts the focus to agency: *your* learning. Generating knowledge requires a relationship between ourselves and our world (Slife & Williams, 1995); that is, *how* we know is shaped by who we are. Our interactions with the world we live in influence, consciously or unconsciously, how we know. These influences include what we observe and take in through our senses (the observable world), our experiences, our previous learning, our culture, our age, our stages of human and professional development, among others.

For example, each of us lives embedded in a culture and cultural groups that define our values and shape our actions. All cultures impose gender-specific work roles: Boys *learn* to do what they *know* men are supposed to do and girls *learn* to do what they *know* women are supposed to do. Culture, thus, profoundly influences how one knows the world (epistemology), what constitutes the reality of that world (ontology), and what are permissible and appropriate actions one can take in that world (norms governing behavior).

To illustrate how life experiences shape our learning, adult development stage theories share some common elements regarding the way we, as humans, view the realities of our worlds: As children we see ourselves as the center and definer of reality; soon we recognize a more dualist view that values the perspectives of authority figures (e.g., parents) over our own; as we grow, we recognize multiple interpretations with reality as relative to a particular context; when we become autonomous, we accept our ability to form our own definitions or interpretations; finally, we learn to integrate our perspectives into a broader, more universal understanding of the world we experience (see, e.g., Belenky, Clinchy, Goldberger, & Tarule, 1997; Levinson, Darrow, & Klein, 1978; Perry, 1970). Thus, how we view the world—our ontology—is shaped by our life development. Similarly, as we grow professionally, we may move through changing foci of interest—from a simple awareness of a concern or problem to a commitment to seek systematic information to improve that problem, and, finally, to taking action.

The link between who we are and how we learn and know must be nurtured to work together if we are to generate knowledge. Bargar and Duncan (1982) assert the importance of the "natural relationships between [the student's] scientific work and her personal and philosophical development, the symbiosis of which creates the deeper psychic perspective essential to original scientific thinking" (p. 4). They refer to the "magic" (p. 4) of challenging personal encounters, and they explore the "experience of scientific invention and its relationship to the self of the scientist" (p. 5).

The point is that wherever we are—developmentally, professionally, experientially, culturally—affects how we see and make sense of, how we know, the world around us. Our way of knowing is our epistemology, our underlying theories of learning; these, in turn, shape what we consider to be the nature, origins, and limits of knowledge (elaborated on in Chapter 2). Thus, inquiry begins with questions *you* want to inform, given your experience and the assumptions you hold of the world. Put simply, we believe that in order to engage in inquiry that will be meaningful to you, tap into your passions and the experiences that have shaped those passions.

DRAWING ON VALUES AND PASSION

Whereas some claim that the scientific method has no room for values or passion, others make a case that science embodies value. Recall the joyful baby scientists (*The Scientist in the Crib*) discussed previously. Certainly, we choose to study what we study for a reason, however convoluted or obscure. James Watson, in *The Double Helix* (1968), on the discovery of DNA, writes: "Science seldom proceeds in the straightforward logical manner imagined by outsiders. Instead, its steps forward (and sometimes backward) are often *very human events in which personalities and cultural traditions* play major roles" (p. ix). He describes a process that required rigorous reasoning but also creativity, politics, mystery, jealousy, and competition. The scientists' passions drove through various iterations of inquiry and eventual discovery of the DNA spiral.

What is your passion?

The story covers the serendipitous journey that brought Watson to join Crick and others in Cambridge, England. At one point, Watson's postdoctoral advisor's marriage was on the rocks, and the advisor was thus "not going to concentrate on science for some time" (1968, p. 25). His advisor's absence left Watson free to bicycle daily to another lab to experiment with the bacterial viruses there. As it progressed, Watson's inquiry process endured near failure (at one point, his superiors ordered that he and Crick give up on DNA) and office tantrums (Watson came near to blows with the cantankerous female crystallographer) through fortuitous detours ("I decided to mark time by working in tobacco mosaic virus" [p. 75]) that culminated in vital discoveries (the tobacco mosaic virus contained the nucleic acid RNA that offered clues to DNA). Throughout, what kept them going was a deep commitment to—their passion for, if you will—making sense of the connections between the various atoms and molecules. Watson admits, "The essential trick was to ask which atoms like to sit next to each other. The main working tools were a set of molecular models superficially resembling the toys of preschool children" (p. 38)—back to the baby scientists.

Indeed, our passion for the subject we study "spurs and guides us" (Polanyi, 1966, p. 75). The intensity with which Barbara McClintock, a Nobel laureate biologist, connected with her corn plants illustrates this passion: She watched each plant to know it intimately, to let it speak to her. "Through a deeply sympathetic understanding, the objects of McClintock's study became subjects in their own right" (Keller, 1983, p. 200). Her goal was to *know* the corn as it is, not as she might imagine it. As Kaplan notes, the "scientific habit of mind is one dominated by the reality principle, by the determination to live in the world as it is and not as we might fantasy it" (1964/2005, p. 147).

Because they are passionate about their searches, scientists do not come to their work value-free. We agree with Becker (1967) that it is simply not possible to do research that is "uncontaminated by personal and political sympathies" (p. 239). "Whatever problems a scientist selects, he selects for a reason and these reasons can be expected to relate to his values or to the values of those who in one way or another influence his choice" (Lundberg & Young, 2005, p. 148). Recall the various influences discussed previously. Values enter into all our choices: the questions we frame, the data we collect, what we determine to be facts (Lundberg & Young, 2005, p. 149). We interpret our findings through the filter of our values. We arrive at information through our interpretation of data—giving something significance or meaning refers to a value. The term *objectivity* takes on a discrete meaning from this perspective: Instead of "value-free," *objectivity* implies "conducted with an open mind." As a value-laden enterprise, however, inquiry demands ethical practice. Ethics—standards for conduct derived from moral principles—guide the scientists' choices, as we discuss in Chapter 4.

YOUR JOURNEY INTO SYSTEMATIC INQUIRY

We hope you are beginning to situate yourself on the journey into meaning making. Becoming an inquiry-minded graduate student is not defined by philosophy or science alone, nor is it a magical mystery tour or a tumble down a rabbit hole. Inquiry is a process that links thinking with doing, theory with practice. Connecting the abstract and the concrete is critical to inquiry, and especially to you as a graduate student. Knowledge is expressed in many and various forms (as we elaborate in Chapter 2), both as ideas and through actions. A theory can stipulate the perceived relationships among a set of concepts bounded by explicit assumptions and limitations or constraints, and thus can provide a clear and helpful way of expressing what we have come to know or what we accept as an understanding or explanation for reality. In short, theories explain interactions among concepts or phenomena. At the same time, our actions also express knowledge. One could say that practice is theory-in-action, that is, a behavioral representation of what we know (see Schön, 1983). Inquiry offers a way to connect what is in our heads with actions. As a graduate student in public policy, for example, you become a social scientist who uses systematic inquiry to connect theories about what people believe should happen (policy) with what people do in programs and practices meant to enact these policies.

This chapter has introduced you to inquiry as an ordinary process people perform every day in a variety of ways. However, as graduate students who are emerging scholars, "the stakes are high . . . [and] your inquiry(ies) will call for a much more conscious, strategic approach" (Brunk-Chavez & Foster, 2010a, p. 2)—*systematic inquiry*, which is a patterned and deliberative process of making decisions about:

Asking "good" questions leads you onward.

- How you will define and frame the focus of the inquiry;
- What will constitute evidence;
- How, where, and from whom you will collect data;
- How you will make sense of the data and the ensuing information; and
- How and with whom you will share or report what you learn.

You will also make decisions about how you document and report the decisions and their rationale so that others may see what you did and why—and may then assess the adequacy of the study and the trustworthiness of the findings.

Through this book, we ask you to take on an *inquiry project*, that is, a project where you, the student, ask critical questions about a topic/issue/ focus/problem of practice. The specific focus of these inquiries may well be what Gunzenhauser and Gerstl-Pepin (2006) call "life-projects"—"the fundamental reasons why graduate students pursue advanced inquiry" (p. 325). This passionate engagement animates your work and your studies. Often, it is the raison d'être for pursuing systematic inquiry. This book is intended to provoke you to consider underlying ideas and assumptions that you bring to this life project and how the issues matter to your professional or everyday world. Although your specific focus may well be a lifetime's work, in this book, we ask you to distill some aspects for sustained inquiry, to carve out a piece of this larger and longer interest to focus on in depth. We have deliberately chosen to use the term *inquiry project* (rather than research study) because the term resonates with principles of inquiry rather than procedures. Toward the end of the book, however, we provide some procedural guidance in developing a research proposal—the encoding of inquiry-in-practice. As well, some of the examples we offer come from students' dissertations and thus represent considerable deeper thinking and work beyond the inquiry project itself.

You will, ultimately, create an argument based on your ideas. We hope to guide you through thought-provoking, sometimes uncomfortable, learning experiences, ones that will strengthen your ability to conceptualize an inquiry project; locate it within "currents of thought" (Schram, 2006, p. 63); critically examine the logic you are building to frame the project; and ask interesting questions that contribute to the project.

The asking of good questions is crucial to any inquiry project. As part of building your own capacities to engage in inquiry that in some way contributes to a larger body of knowledge, you will come to look critically at claims other authors make, weigh and assess the evidence they put forward, and see logical flaws in their arguments. We hope that you will learn to read "against the grain" (Regaignon, 2009, p. 124), which, in turn, will help you critically read your own writings and those of your community of practice.

We bring to this book a set of our own assumptions about inquiry and inquirers:

- Inquiry involves ongoing processes of learning about the world, how it works, and how it can be changed;
- Systematic inquiry is a process of conceptualizing, designing, conducting, documenting, and reporting what is learned;

- Critical feedback, reflection, and modification are essential to inquiry and knowledge generation;
- The inquirer is a learner, continually and consciously making decisions that affect the questions pursued and the direction of the inquiry;
- The learner is central to his or her own learning and is responsible for it;
- Each learner constructs knowledge in his or her own way according to individual experiences, gender, abilities, style, language, and preferences; and
- The products of inquiry, in whatever form they take, should be used to improve the human condition.

We confess that our conceptualization of and the corollary assumptions about inquiry are inspired by and grounded in the many writings of John Dewey, an American philosopher of the 20th century. His ideas on the indeterminateness of knowledge and on the interaction between experience and reflection as ground for knowledge construction have deeply shaped our own learning and teaching.

Inquiry, then, mediates curiosity and observations through the learner's experiences, cultural orientation, developmental stage, learning style preferences, personality, and so on and on. Ultimately, inquiry is *not* about proving something, not about establishing certainty. Instead, inquiry—that is, learning—is heuristic, a discovery of possibilities and potential answers or solutions, albeit temporary, ephemeral, and context bound. To understand inquiry, we briefly explore ways of knowing and forms that knowledge may take or be expressed in, and consider how humans systematize inquiry.

Learning Activity 1.1. "Nanook of the North"

We offer this learning experience to invite you to see that there are multiple, sometimes conflicting, ways of understanding an event or circumstance. In our classes, we show the opening scene from the video *Nanook of the North*, a classic anthropological film depicting an event from life of the Inuit in the 1920s. The scene shows Nanook paddling his canoe up to land and getting out of it. Several other persons exit from the canoe; we stop the film after the last one has exited.

In your group, watch this key excerpt from the video twice and then ask, "What is going on here? What do you see?" Invite as many responses as possible as a brainstorming activity (no comment, no judgments). Once many responses have been offered, shift to the question, "How do you know?" In our classes, we refer to a few specific responses, asking those students to elaborate, to tease out what their "evidence" is for their ideas. We then ask, "What more would you like to know?" and "How might you go about getting that?" Consider asking similar probing questions in your group.

The purpose of this activity is to surface a range of interpretations of what is (actually) going on. We have found that it leads to lively discussions, sometimes quite heated, about what the video depicts. The main point is often best left unsaid: that there are multiple views/interpretations of one scene or set of circumstances, and that we really cannot be sure is what "actually" happening.

Learning Activity 1.2. Problematizing "Truth"

This activity can serve to illustrate the links between individual and social construction of knowledge. Start by thinking of something *you know to be true*. Then relate this "truth" to the person next to you. Together, critique the "truth": Is it always true? Under what circumstances? Would everyone agree that this is true? Why or why not? When did you learn or decide this truth? How do you know? What evidence can you offer?

As a large group, debrief the conversations, using ideas presented in this chapter, such as Scheffler's criteria, relationships between who we are and what we know and value, the concept of *Homo sapiens sapiens*, and assumptions about learning and inquiry.

FOR FURTHER READING

➥ Blaikie, N. (2007). *Approaches to social enquiry* (2nd ed.). Cambridge, UK: Polity Press.

➥ Berger, P. L., & Luckmann, T. (1967). *The social construction of reality: A treatise in the sociology of knowledge.* New York: Anchor Books, Doubleday.

➥ Brady, H. E., & Collier, D. (Eds.). (2010). *Rethinking social inquiry: Diverse tools, shared standards* (2nd ed.). Lanham, MD: Rowman & Littlefield.

Cooper, F., & Packard, R. (Eds.). (1997). *International development and the social sciences: Essays on the history and politics of knowledge.* Berkeley: University of California Press.

Flyvbjerg, B. (2001). *Making social science matter: Why social inquiry fails and how it can succeed again.* Cambridge, UK: Cambridge University Press.

King, G., & Keohane, R. O. (1994). *Designing social inquiry: Scientific inference in qualitative research.* Princeton, NJ: Princeton University Press.

Lundberg, C. C., & Young, C. A. (Eds.). (2005). *Foundations for inquiry: Choices and trade-offs in the organizational sciences.* Stanford, CA: Stanford Business Books.

McMillan, J., & Schumacher, S. (2006). *Research in education: Evidence-based inquiry* (6th ed.). Boston: Pearson/Allyn & Bacon.

Phillips, D. C. (2006). A guide for the perplexed: Scientific educational research, methodolatry, and the gold versus platinum standards. *Educational Research Review, 1,* 15–26.

Reason, P. (1981). *Human inquiry: A sourcebook of new paradigm research.* Wiley.

CHAPTER 2

Ways of Knowing
Finding a Compass

❋ *Critical Questions to Guide Your Reading*

➥ *What are key philosophies about knowing? (remembering)*

➥ *How do these compare with one another? (analyzing)*

➥ *What are ontology and epistemology? (remembering)*

➥ *How do assumptions within these philosophical fields shape my approach to inquiry? (applying)*

➥ *What is my theory of social change? (applying)*

➥ *How does this theory inform my approach to inquiry? (applying)*

Dialogue 2. What Do We Know? How Do We Know It?

Students in Professor Bettara's *Inquiry* class are sitting in small groups. Bettara has asked them to make a statement of something they know about an issue or topic that they are interested in. In turn, they are to share their "assertions"; the other members of the group then ask questions to clarify and encourage elaboration.

KEVIN: OK. I'll start. I think this assignment seems pretty straightforward—I like that. What I would say is that, from my experience

19

in schools, principals are absolutely critical for a successful school culture.

RAUL: First salvo is mine! Kevin, just what do you mean by "critical"? "Essential"? That a school won't have a successful culture without a principal? Another thought: Does just any principal do this? Or does a principal have to do certain things?

MARTINA: Thanks for being brave and starting, Kevin. Now, my question is about what you mean by a "successful school culture"? I've heard that idea a lot, but I'm not sure what you mean by it. Can you tell us what it looks like? Is what's successful in one place successful in another? I'm thinking about Kenya now, where it would certainly be different! There, success might be defined by access, especially for the girl child. Any thoughts? Or are these too many questions?

REILLY: Now it's my turn. Kevin, you'll get a chance to respond soon! I think that you need to use a more postmodern . . . you know, a power lens to look at the principal and culture, like who gets to say what "culture" is? You know from McTaggart's class that there's a lot written about how "the powerful" define success and then they impose that definition on everyone else, like the so-called "marginalized." So I'd suggest you think about that. Another thought: Haven't principals been studied a lot already? So what's the point?

SAMIRA: I like that, Reilly. Power might be a really important idea for what Kevin wants to study. But "postmodern" and "marginalized" sound like jargon. And I'd guess that's part of Kevin's perspective; he's just not using those terms. Kevin, do you want to look at the principal as a power position? Wait! Don't answer just yet. Because what I take from what you've said is that you really want to explore the role of the principal, whatever that may be, and how these folks help schools be successful, yes? And I sense that what you claim to know about the importance of the principal comes from your own experience . . . you are a principal, right?

KEVIN: Yes, at the vocational high school. And before that—

REILLY: (*interrupting*) But how do you know principals are so important? Don't you think that there's a lot more to know than just your
own experience? I'd say it's a lot more complex than that. And anyway, are all principals like you?

RAUL: Good points. Could have been said more gently. Sorry for that,
Kevin. But it seems that you need to be careful about thinking that
your experience tells you what things are like in other schools.
Case in point: Last year I was subbing in schools after I left my job
on Wall Street, and all I ever saw principals do was hold meetings
and walk the halls picking up paper. But my experience is just that.
Not yours and not everyone else's. So, I wonder how we can *ever*
say we know something. Can we ever be certain? It's a bit scary to
keep asking "how" we know anything!

SAMIRA: Kevin, I'm not sure this has been at all helpful. Has it? I'll bet
you have a lot to think about, but remember that we're with you!

KEVIN: Wow. Thanks. I still "know" the principal is important, but your
questions remind me how complicated it is. Can we put someone
else in "the hot seat"? Martina, you ready?

Their group dialogue explores and critiques the various statements of
each member. What becomes clear is the complexity and problematic
nature of what anyone labels as knowledge.

As this dialogue reveals, Professor Bettara's students are beginning to consider—and articulate—how they know what they know about topics they
may want to explore further. First, let us introduce our characters:

Martina, who is from Kenya, is concerned about the effects of health
problems on children in her country. Specifically, she has seen many
HIV/AIDS orphans, some as young as 10 years, assume roles as head of
household. As well, her experiences with colonial occupation make her
critical of Western intervention. She has come to graduate school because
she hopes her learning and advanced degree will empower her to make
changes in her country's public health and social systems.

Raul, who worked for a large international banking firm, became disillusioned with the dollar-driven ethics of the financial workplace. After dropping out of his Wall Street job, he spent a year as a substitute teacher in the New York City public schools. Having experienced two contrasting worlds (finance and education), he has returned to the university for a degree in management. He hopes that learning organizational theory and behavior will help him bridge the two worlds and find a means of improving both. His background has taught him to identify and build clear and logical arguments, while his creativity causes him to question the status quo.

Kevin has been an urban high school principal for a decade. His reasons for seeking a doctorate in educational administration are pragmatic; the degree will give him status and security—and he wants answers to problems he encounters in his work. Uncomfortable with ambiguity, his views are practical and dualist; he sees the world primarily in black and white. Tired because he is always working, Kevin comes late to class and rarely gets engaged in an issue or problem unless he can relate to it personally or professionally. He arrives with a traditional interest in the principalship but becomes intrigued with exploring the learning challenges adolescent boys experience as they enter high school—and the role principals may play in supporting boys' learning.

Samira is sensitive to the emotions and needs of others, as evidenced in her demonstrated commitment to social justice. She has spent the past 8 years as an organizer/activist in an extremely poor rural community and has become troubled by the failure of the community's youth to persist in getting higher education degrees. As a graduate student, she seeks to understand the connections among public policy, programs, and practice, specifically, what institutional policies support or hinder access and persistence. Always practical, she asks: How's this going to play on the ground?

Reilly has never held a full-time job; he went directly from undergraduate to graduate school, receiving a master's degree in sociology and political science, without a break. Now he is entering a doctoral program. At this point, he is quick to critique others but seldom questions his own ideas or assertions. A perennial graduate student, he draws heavily on theory, and in nearly every comment he refers to Marx or neoliberalism or critical theory. He plans to become a professor.

The specific purpose of Dialogue 2 is to depict the central challenges of examining what you claim to know and how you know it. As our students demonstrate, simply saying what you know is not as easy or straightforward as it may seem. They raise several important points: for example, how does Kevin define the terms he uses ("critical," "successful school culture")? What alternative opinions/views might other people hold? What is already known about the importance of a principal, based on previous research? Do theoretical lenses exist to help Kevin understand the principal's role in relation to other roles? How does Kevin's experience as a principal influence what he knows? Finally, how can Kevin know what he knows, and how can he claim that he knows?

This chapter explores answers to these questions. We first discuss varying ways of knowing; then we present some assumptions about ways of knowing and about the social world; and we end the chapter with some strategies for thinking about your own perspective on inquiry. Who you are as an inquirer is shaped by your experiences, what you learn, what you value, and how you hope to engage with your topic.

WAYS OF KNOWING

As mentioned in Chapter 1, each of us holds assumptions about what makes up reality (ontology) and how that reality can be known (epistemology). These assumptions are grounded in who we are and how we learn. Various perspectives or paradigmatic beliefs about ontology have developed that establish scholarly conceptualizations of what is taken as reality. Similarly, scholars over the centuries and across cultures have presented multiple epistemologies that offer some philosophical foundations for knowing reality. At the risk of glossing over their more complex meanings, we present several models to help you begin to locate your own beliefs and to analyze and understand your ways of knowing. You may note that we begin with Western thinkers because we know those best; however, we do refer to non-Western models and encourage you to explore them more fully. Most important, we suggest that anyone's way of knowing does not formulaically follow just one of the models but is actually a synthesis of several models. We acknowledge that our interpretaions of these philosophers' ideas are somewhat superficial and incomplete, especially those with non-Western traditions, and that we are condensing into a few pages what others have devoted volumes to. Still, our purpose is to provide historical context. We hope the following synopses serve to pique your interest, and we encourage you to explore more deeply and directly those that interest you.

• *Plato* (c. 424–348 B.C.E.), through Socrates, offered an early epistemological model. He presented knowledge as a product of reasoning, the *Socratic method* of questioning to uncover a logical reasoning that yields answers. Socratic questioning facilitates "discovery" of answers within oneself. Knowledge resides within us; as humans, we all drink from the river of knowledge, so learning is a process of surfacing the knowledge we need at any given time. For example, when we see a horse, we recognize that specific animal as a horse because an image or reflection of "horse" already exists in our mind. Knowing is concept driven, or deductive; we start with ideas that generate details. The way to know is through reasoning, not direct experience, which cannot be trusted because experiences themselves are reflections of reality.

• *Aristotle* (384–322 B.C.E.), although a student of Plato, posited, quite differently, that knowledge is available only through our sensory experiences of the external world. Knowing is, thus, data driven. We observe, we make sense of our observations, we know. The process is inductive, the opposite of Plato's; we start with the details and construct the whole. The reality of "horse" comes from the details we see—the mane, the hoof, the leg—our observations combine to build the whole.

• Jumping centuries, we find *John Locke* (1632–1704), who combined experience and reason. He asserted that your mind is born *tabula rasa* (blank slate) on which experiences etch representations of the external world. Your reflections on these experiences yield interpretations or constructed meanings (thus qualifying Locke as an early constructivist because he described how an individual constructs his or her world).

• *Behavioralists*, such as *B. F. Skinner* (1904–1990) and *Ivan Pavlov* (1849–1936), viewed learning as conditioning. Their conceptualization drew upon both Aristotle and Locke: Experiences, which include stimuli, shape our behaviors; we learn to generalize across stimuli.

• Rejecting the tabula rasa perspective, *Immanuel Kant* (1724–1804) pictured our minds as responding to both sensory perception and reason. What we see or experience is shaped by who we are and the context in which we see or experience; at the same time, the object or experience shapes the context and who we are. For example, time, space, and physical structure are some conditions that influence what we see and how we experience the world. However, when reason and sensory experience fail to provide answers, humans turn to an innate universal moral law, that is, one that holds authority in all cases for all people. According to Kant, we use this moral law unconsciously, as a moral compass or guide for deciding what is right or wrong.

• *Jean Piaget* (1896–1980) elaborated the importance of growth and development in how we know. He demonstrated how we progress through stages that define our epistemology. We move from states of *equilibrium*, that is, stages of certainty about our knowing, through *disequilibrium*, which challenges that certainty, to new stages of equilibrium. These, in turn, will be challenged as we grow. Thus, knowing is a process of construction and reconstruction triggered by cognitive growth.

• *Lev Vygotsky* (1896–1934), who also adhered to the stage, or developmental, theory, added the social aspect of learning. His construct of *zones of proximal development* describes how children learn while interacting with other children who are at slightly more advanced stages of knowing. As a Western thinker who lived and wrote under that Soviet regime that emphasized the collective, Vygotsky eases us toward some non-Western epistemologies that view knowledge as a group or community commodity. For example, many African communities, such as the Bantu people of southern Africa, view human existence in relation to the existence of others; that is, "a person is because of others" (Chilisa, 2009, p. 413). From this perspective, knowledge is communal, collective, and plural.

• Our consideration of epistemological models would hardly be complete without mention of two eastern philosophies. The *Taoist tradition* (*Tao Te Ching*, Lao-tse, fifth–fourth century B.C.E.) recognizes a mystical source of all being. The *Dao* emphasizes harmony, presence, and balance; we know by attending to and accepting the present moment as a natural state. What is, is and does not need explication. In contrast, *Confucius* (551–479 B.C.E.) reminds us that knowledge comes from long and careful study of the past, respecting elders and family authority; knowledge is learning that integrates experiences. Thus, we learn through analysis and synthesis of the past.

This brief overview can be used to identify various ways knowledge can be used. For example, knowledge can be seen as:

- *Propositional*—describes or declares what is known;
- *Procedural*—tells how, and especially how best, to perform some task; and/or
- *Principled*—reveals understanding the comprehensive and fundamental laws, doctrines, or assumptions underlying an idea or activity.

To illustrate, take knowledge about cooking. First, the cook or someone in the setting proposes an idea or plan for the meal; this proposition requires knowledge of possibilities as well as a means for articulating the suggestion. Next, the cook needs procedures for preparing the meal; these usually take the form of recipes. A truly experienced cook, however, knows the patterns of the procedures so well that he may not need the recipe (or may alter it) because he understands the principles that underlie the procedures. Specifically, someone may propose that you make bread: "We need fresh bread to spread with butter and dip into the soup." If your knowledge of bread making is procedural, you will find and follow a recipe. Perhaps you understand how flour binds with liquid and eggs, rises with yeast or soda, and bakes, and can be flavored. Because you have principled knowledge, you mix and knead and find heat; you don't need a recipe. Of course, you might point out that the mere knowledge of how to make bread is inconsequential compared with the knowledge of how great bread tastes (a sensory form of knowledge)!

These different ways people use to describe knowledge reveal the complexity and multiplicity of human understanding of *knowing*. Many other descriptions are available, including:

- *Practical*—we know what works;
- *Experiential*—we know from doing;
- *Observational*—we know from watching;
- *Rational*—we know through reasoning; and
- *Discursive*—we know dialogically, through talking with and testing ideas out with others.

A useful way to view knowledge may be captured in a definition of intelligence: "the capacity to solve problems or to fashion products that are valued in one or more cultural setting" (Gardner & Hatch, 1989, p. 5). From this definition, Howard Gardner argued that traditional definitions of intelligence were not sufficient to cover the range of abilities needed to solve problems or create products that could be valued or found useful in various settings. For example, while schools value skill in writing and math, baseball players value the ability to use their bodies to hit the ball, and those attending a rock concert would value the skill of the drummer to perform.

Gardner (1993, 1999) identifies three sets of intelligences that can be considered to be *ways of knowing*: linguistic and logical-mathematical (valued in school); musical, bodily-kinesthetic, and spatial (valued in the arts and sports); and intrapersonal and interpersonal (valued in relationships). While each way of knowing can be drawn on separately, they often interact and complement each other. His theory of multiple intelligences supports the existence of multiple ways of knowing.

You may note that each expression of knowledge is, in a sense, an inquiry: We discover through describing, doing, watching, reasoning, playing, dreaming, talking. According to Dewey (1938), inquiry is the tool that serves discovery, that is, the investigation and solution to the problems of humans. The point and purpose of inquiry are to be found in (1) the interconnectedness between inquiry and (2) the situation in which it is used and in its capacity to serve the use goals of growth and of the community. The specific context of the inquiry recognizes the relevant data points that build the information. As well, it is the context in which the information rests that facilitates use. Epistemological, experiential, logical, and aesthetic concerns all have a place in inquiry (see Figure 2.1).

To help students grapple with these ideas, we engage them in several perspective-changing learning activities (see Learning Activities 2.2 and

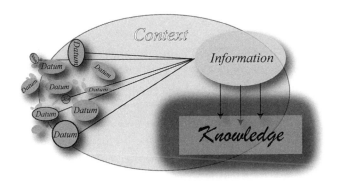

FIGURE 2.1. Data, information, knowledge, and context.

2.3 found at the end of the chapter). Our purpose is to unfreeze (see Lewin, 1951) routine and habitual ways of seeing the world.

FUNDAMENTAL ASSUMPTIONS

The previous chapter and its learning activities illustrate that inquiry is informed by fundamental understandings about the nature of reality, what human nature is, how human beings interact with their environment, the social world, and how we come to know all of this and make claims about what we have learned in an inquiry project.

> Epistemology?
> Ontology?

Exploring these understandings helps to clarify your perspective—your "intellectual orientation" (Schram, 2006, pp. 40–52)—as you undertake a project. This exploration is crucial for locating and understanding where you stand—your orientation—relative to the work you want to undertake. This assertion has implications for *what* you focus on to learn more about, *how* you come to know that world more deeply, and the relevance of what you learn to your world and others'. And this assertion captures important ideas that philosophers and research methodologists grapple with. This orientation is also described as your *stance*, your *perspective*, or the *paradigm* where you situate yourself. While the term *paradigm* has been used to capture this cluster of assumptions, we find it "overworked, overused, and trivialized" (Rossman & Rallis, 2012, p. 35) and prefer the terms *orientation* and *perspective*; we use these interchangeably.

What makes up "orientation"? Philosophers of science have argued that one's orientation is formed by sets of deep assumptions one holds, perhaps unconsciously. The first set is assumptions about reality, the nature of human existence, and how human beings interact with their environments; this is called *ontology*, as we have mentioned before. The second set captures assumptions about what knowledge really is, what is accepted as knowledge claims, and what is taken as evidence; this is one's *epistemology*. These sets of assumptions, then, shape how one goes about conceiving and implementing an inquiry project; this is the preferred *methodology*, which is shaped by ontological and epistemological assumptions.

Given that we are writing to an audience in the social sciences and applied fields, however, it is also crucial to reflect on and examine the assumptions we make about the social, rather than the natural, world.

Ontology, epistemology, and methodology are philosophically based concepts. We try to make them more clear next.

Ontological Assumptions

As it has evolved over the years, the philosophical branch of ontology grapples with questions about existence, the self, and what constitutes reality. What is the nature of existence? Who am I? What is reality? And how do I interact with that reality/environment as a bodied self? To help get clear about your assumptions about the nature of reality and human existence, ask yourself the following questions. The questions represent binaries that force you to consider extreme positions; you realize that an answer could be: "It depends...." Note that these questions have implications for how you would come to know that reality (your epistemology).

- Do I believe that reality is of an objective nature? Does reality exist independently of my perception, as something "out there" that I can learn about without direct experience?
- Is reality the product of my individual and social experiences? Do I create or co-create reality? (Adapted from Rossman & Rallis, 2012, p. 38)

Also subsumed under this set of assumptions are those we make about the nature of human agency—that is, how and in what ways human beings use their capacity to choose and act efficaciously in the world. Recall the earlier mention of the learner's agency. Again, we raise a set of binary questions:

- Do I assume that people respond to forces without much ability to change them? Or do people themselves influence or construct the forces?
- Are we shaped by external circumstances? Or do we shape those circumstances?
- Do we assume human action is predetermined? Or do we have the free will to make the path we walk on?
- Do we see situations as more or less stable? Or do we see situations as continually changing? (Adapted from Rossman & Rallis, 2012, p. 39)

Epistemological Assumptions

Some of the notions discussed previously in the Ways of Knowing section introduced the key ideas that are subsumed under epistemology. To repeat, central are questions about what constitutes truth and what I mean when I say I know something. To clarify your assumptions about epistemology, ask yourself:

- How do I know that I know something?
- What do I take as truth?
- What convinces me of the credibility of a claim that something is true?
- What do I take as evidence to support a point?
- Do I tend to accept what I read and hear, or am I a bit skeptical, asking critical questions before accepting? (Adapted from Rossman & Rallis, 2012, p. 37)
- How do I learn something?
- What do I believe is the appropriate relationship between the knower and the known?

As we shall see, epistemological and ontological assumptions are interrelated. If I believe that only one objective social reality exists, I would be likely to seek an authority to tell me. On the other hand, if I believe that there are multiple social realities, I would talk with other people.

Methodological Assumptions

Assumptions held—whether consciously or not—in the domains just mentioned have implications for how one approaches and conducts an inquiry project. If the assumptions are more objectivist, the project will likely rely on randomization and the power of large-scale predictive statistical analysis. If, on the other hand, the assumptions are more interpretive, the project will likely be designed to get close to people, learning directly from them about their experiences. These orientations—objectivist and interpretivist—are discussed more fully shortly.

Assumptions about the Social World

Also relevant for exploring one's intellectual perspective are assumptions about the nature of the social world. At issue here is the model or working understanding about how social structures and processes work in the world. Tendencies are for an emphasis on orderly change, regulated and predictable processes, or for an emphasis on oppression and domination. If the assumptions about the social world tend toward orderly change, the inquiry project will likely seek greater understanding and perhaps improvement of some set of circumstances. If, however, assumptions tend toward those viewing social forces as dominating and oppressive, the project may be inclined toward questions and outcomes that might radically alter circumstances—for the better.

MAPPING PERSPECTIVES

To pull these sets of assumptions together, we refer to the work, now 40 years old and still generative, of Burrell and Morgan (1979), sociologists who described two sets of continua and four paradigms to provide a heuristic for exploring your assumptions. As noted previously, we prefer the terms *orientation* or *perspective* but defer to their use of *paradigm* in this discussion.

The first continuum describes ontological, epistemological, and methodological assumptions along an objectivist–subjectivist axis. Again, we gently critique the term *subjectivist* and have substituted *interpretivist* as a less value-laden term; we use our preferred term in this discussion (see Rossman & Rallis, 2012, pp. 43–44). The second continuum describes assumptions about the nature of the social world; this is the sociology of regulation–sociology of radical change axis.

The Objectivist–Interpretivist Continuum

This continuum describes a range of assumptions you may hold about the nature of reality and about knowledge and knowing. At one extreme anchor point are objectivist assumptions that posit reality to be pretty much independent of social actors; generating knowledge about that reality is fact based. At the other extreme are interpretivist assumptions that view reality as socially constructed and laden with multiple meanings; learning about

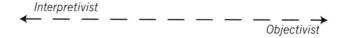

FIGURE 2.2. The interpretivist–objectivist continuum.

that reality is fruitfully accomplished through direct personal experience. These are depicted in Figure 2.2 above.

The implications of various positions on this continuum for your inquiry project may well be profound. More interpretivist assumptions lend themselves toward face-to-face interactions and may well draw on dreams, memories, poems, and other evocative discourse to construct an understanding of social phenomena. More objectivist assumptions would encourage an inquirer to remain objective in an inquiry project, to rely on distance and instrumentation in order to generate findings about the phenomenon of interest. Developed by Evered and Louis some years ago (1981) but still useful is the distinction between "inquiry from the inside" and "inquiry from the outside" (p. 385).

The Sociology of Regulation–Sociology of Radical Change Continuum

Also relevant, since your inquiry projects will focus on some aspect of the social world, are assumptions you make about social processes—that is, how the social world(s) work and how social structures and processes change. Do you tend to think that social processes are, in essence, orderly? Predictable? Changeable but only over time and slowly? In contrast, your assumptions about and experiences of social processes might draw you to see the social world as essentially conflictual, oppressive, characterized by domination and power. These notions might lead you to think that social change must be radical, transformative.

For example, your area of interest may be early childhood literacy. For your inquiry project, your purpose may be to learn why some children learn to read early and others later. You hope that what you discover may inform curriculum and instruction in schools. Alternatively, your interest may be in young children's access to reading materials and opportunities; your intent may be to eventually change the social and economic circumstances that limit some children's access. Each study would map differently on the continua (see Figure 2.3).

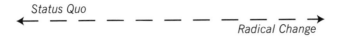

FIGURE 2.3. The status quo–radical change continuum.

To help students begin to get in touch with these sets of assumptions—not the sort of questions we go about asking in a typical day—we have developed Learning Activity 2.3 (at the end of the chapter) to help make these questions real. As you engage in this activity, you'll see that the two continua interact, suggesting your particular intellectual orientation and your assertions regarding your topic of interest. For example, Kevin believes that the school principal is important to increasing student learning, and that the principal's role can change and improve. He may see the role of the school principal as independent of the person in the role and the specific school, and thus might argue that we need to define clearly a model in which all principals should be trained in order to bring about positive reform in schools. In contrast, Kevin may see the role as defined by the context of the individual school and the personal characteristics of that principal; from this view, he would argue that understanding how different principals define and enact their roles in their various contexts would lead to multiple approaches for a principal to support school improvement. In each case, he would locate himself at different places on the continua.

BACK TO ONTOLOGY AND EPISTEMOLOGY

We have invited you to consider *ways of knowing* by introducing the ontological and epistemological foundations of inquiry and differentiating between various theoretical models and modes of inquiry: What is knowledge? How is knowledge generated? How does knowledge affect practice? Who uses knowledge and in what ways? To what ends?

We recognize that ontology and epistemology represent complex concepts, but they capture important ideas: ways we view the world, ways we interact with one another, what we accept as true, what we accept as evidence (what convinces us). These are knotty concepts, but we try to move into them directly, reminding you that feeling some discomfort is often a good thing. Learning theorists have written about how upsetting one's habitual ways of thinking can be quite generative. Concepts like "unfreezing"

(Lewin, 1951) and "disequilibrium" (Piaget, 1953) capture this idea. Argyris (1993) asserts that we learn best when we encounter mismatches, when our routine notions are upset. Piaget (1953) describes how crucial this process of upsetting existing ideas—disequilibration—is for doing the hard work of building new knowledge and skills. Vygotsky (1978) argues that experiences in the zone of proximal development encourage learning and growth. And don't forget that baby—the scientist in the crib—who experiments with and learns from puzzles in his or her surrounding world.

You may find comfort in narrowing the ideas around ontology and epistemology to the general area you want to study for your project, or you might get more stressed if you have no idea yet for the project. Just remember that the purpose of this book is to guide you through the inquiry process, specifically academic inquiry regarding a research project. In summary, what we claim to know is a result of a complicated interaction between the knower and the known. Our values and interests and ethics—passions and principles—are part of who we are and thus play a major role in determining or generating what we say we know. We bring them to any and all inquiry, whether it be scientific and systematic or personal and informal. In the next chapter, we start you on your way by introducing the inquiry cycle with various models of inquiry in practice.

Learning Activity 2.1. The Magic Eye®

For this activity, we provide several images from the Magic Eye (*www. magiceye.com*). If you are not familiar with them, these are three-dimensional images that invite alternative ways of seeing. They are "ranked" from easier to harder to "see." We follow the instructions on the Magic Eye website below:

> Hold the center of the printed image *right up to your nose*. It should be blurry. Focus as though you are looking *through* the image into the distance. *Very slowly* move the image away from your face until the *two squares* above the image turn into *three squares*. If you see four squares, move the image farther away from your face until you see three squares. If you see one or two squares, start over!

When you clearly see three squares, hold the page still, and the hidden image will magically appear. Once you perceive the hidden image and depth, you can look around the entire 3-D image. The longer you look, the clearer the illusion becomes. The farther away you hold the page, the deeper it becomes (*www.magiceye.com/faq_example.htm*).

We always have several images available, and we raise questions such as: How easy was it for you to see the alternative image? Were you surprised? If you were unable to see the image, what did it feel like not to be able to see what someone else saw? For those who did see the image, what were the challenges in trying to explain what you saw to someone who was unable to see what you did? We remind you that everyone in the group is looking at the same object.

Learning Activity 2.2. Alternative Maps

Yet another learning activity helps you experience very different ways of viewing the world through maps. The purpose here is to help you see that deeply held views are often quite limited, shaped by culture and socialization; they represent what we are accustomed to seeing.

ODT, Inc., located in Amherst, Massachusetts, produces "alternative maps" that depict the world in ways other than the standard Mercator projection. Examples include the "What's Up? South!" map, which challenges our perceived notions of "up" and "down" by placing south at the top of the map. Another is a world population map, which depicts the size of countries based on their populations. In this map, China and India are quite large, whereas Europe is quite small. (See *http://odtmaps.com* for details on these and other maps.) We show these maps in our classes to invite students to consider how these alternative representations challenge their assumptions about the world. We suggest that you and your classmates look over such maps and discuss your reactions. Rallis has had these maps tacked to her wall for several years, and she has noticed how students have grown so accustomed to seeing them that they are "reality." They will gesture to indicate what country they are from, as if these were "standard" maps.

Learning Activity 2.3. Strings

To enact and embody the ideas of continua described in this chapter, we bring to class long strings or twine of two different colors, which we attach to the east–west and north–south sides of the classroom. We suggest you try this activity with your classmates. See Figure 2.4.

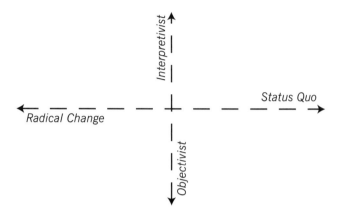

FIGURE 2.4. Four paradigms.

Name one as the *objectivist–interpretivist* continuum and indicate which end represents which set of assumptions. Then place yourselves somewhere you feel you belong along the string. This typically involves much chatter and laughter and even questions like "Why are you there, Samira?" Follow with a short debriefing, asking volunteers to explain why they situated themselves where they did and to consider under which conditions they might place themselves somewhere else.

Next name the other string as the *status quo–radical change* continuum and now move to where you feel most comfortable. Again, follow with a debriefing; now the questions focus on how the two continua interact to affect your placement. What does it mean, for example, to be standing near the objectivist end but also close to the radical change end? Again, consider how your positionality might change depending on the focus and purpose of what you are doing or thinking about.

FOR FURTHER READING

↪ Bateson, G. (2002). *Mind and nature: A necessary unity*. Cresskill, NJ: Hampton Press.

↪ Blumer, H. (1969). *Symbolic interaction*. Englewood Cliffs, NJ: Prentice-Hall. See pp. 78–89.

↪ Burrell, G., & Morgan, G. (1979). *Sociological paradigms and organizational analysis*. London: Heinemann.

Crumley, J. S. (1998). *Introduction to epistemology.* Mountain View, CA: Mayfield.

Harris, M. (Ed.). (2007). *Ways of knowing: New approaches in the anthropology of knowledge and learning.* Oxford, UK: Berghan Books.

Phillips, D. C. (1985). On what scientists know, and how they know it. In E. Eisner (Ed.), *Learning and teaching the ways of knowing: The 84th Yearbook of the National Society for the Study of Education* (pp. 37–59). Chicago: University of Chicago Press.

Schratz, M., & Walker, R. (1995). *Research as social change: New opportunities for qualitative research.* London: Routledge.

Slife, B. D., & Williams, R. N. (1995). *What's behind the research?: Discovering hidden assumptions in the behavioral sciences.* Thousand Oaks, CA: Sage.

CHAPTER 3

The Cycle of Inquiry
More Than One Way to Get There

⚙ *Critical Questions to Guide Your Reading*

→ *What are the key elements of cycles of inquiry? (remembering)*

→ *How do theories of learning and inquiry relate to one another? (analyzing)*

→ *What aspects of cycles of inquiry are relevant for my inquiry project? (applying)*

→ *What makes a study trustworthy? (remembering)*

→ *How can I integrate strategies to help my study be credible? (applying)*

→ *Which considerations of trustworthiness best suit my project? (evaluating)*

Dialogue 3. Conducting Inquiry: How Do I Do It?

Students in Professor Bettara's *Inquiry* class are again sitting in small groups: They have been asked to talk about how they came to know their assertion.

SAMIRA: I have to tell you, for maybe the first time in my schooling I'm hearing something I am comfortable with—that knowledge is not definite. That it isn't just what sits on the shelves over in the library. That I actually can, in fact *do*, create it.

RAUL: Yeah, I agree. I've always really hated being told that someone knows the truth! All I need to do is follow a story on the web, and I can see it just keeps changing, even hourly. Even what passes for research can tell different stories. So how do people make sense of all that's out there?

KEVIN: How can you both feel that way? I mean, doesn't the uncertainty make you nervous? If we have a problem, how can we know what is right, what will work? I'm thinking about my students' test scores, the achievement gap—I want answers on what will help them improve!

MARTINA: I think I know what you mean, Kevin. I want answers too, but I don't want answers that were developed for privileged families in the USA. I want "knowledge" that will work for the situation in Kenya. Bettara mentioned "systematic inquiry," but I wonder what different ways to create knowledge exist.

REILLY: I'm with you on that—that's the power issue I talked about last time. Is Bettara going to impose some "gold standard" inquiry method on us?

KEVIN: Well, I for one hope so. I don't want to waste my time doing some inquiry project that won't tell me anything I can use in my school. I thought that the definition of knowledge included use. And that's just what I need!

SAMIRA: Settle down, you two. I think you've missed the point of last week's class—that we play a big part in defining what we know. Didn't you hear Bettara refer to an "inquiry cycle"? My guess is that if it's a cycle, there's more than one way to do it.

KEVIN: OK. So what's the process? Do I begin with a question or a problem? I've got both of those. Then what do I do?

RAUL: I doubt it's that simple. Maybe the question I have doesn't get at the real problem, so I have to do some pre-question thinking. And while I agree that each of us shapes what we know, so do the worlds we live in. Like, scientists use something called the scientific method. How does that mesh with inquiry cycles, like that teachers use to solve problems in classrooms? I'm pretty sure they don't use the same inquiry cycle that my banker colleagues—or the stockbrokers—used on Wall Street!

KEVIN: Talk about uncertainty!

REILLY: Power again. So obviously there's more than one way to do this. Which ways are legitimate? Credible? Get the "stamp of approval"?

MARTINA: What's important to me is that, whatever the inquiry cycle is, I can actually do it. I mean, it's got to be practical. A lot of families in villages in Kenya have children who are heads of households because the parents have died from AIDS. I need to know more about these families. So many questions that I don't know where to begin. And I won't have a lot of resources, so I'll have to do it myself. I've heard enough theory; I want to hear how I can do this so it's practical.

INQUIRY IN ACTION/INQUIRY AS PRACTICE

So far, we have been talking a lot about inquiry. You have read that inquiry is a natural but often complex, even ambiguous, learning process to make sense of the world. Either formally or informally, inquiry brings together data in various forms to build information; through our individual and social lenses, we interpret and use this information as knowledge. We have considered that inquiry links thinking with doing. As a naturally occurring set of activities, each cycle involves: a trigger → questions → immersion (research) → incubation (letting it cook) → insight (aha!) → communicating and testing the information → using it as knowledge. While on paper the process appears to be linear and sequential, in practice it is iterative and cyclical, one activity building on another with a lot of recycling back. As Dewey (1896) reminds us, both experiencing and thinking about the experience are essential; thus, a form of inquiry is embedded in every step. Furthermore, the process is interpretive (even numbers must be interpreted), with the inquirer making sense along the way. Finally, it is heuristic—a discovery.

Inquiry = curiosity.

Yet we have not presented inquiry as a practice. Now let's look at examples of inquiry in action: What do people actually do as they engage in cycles of inquiry? You may be familiar with one or more models for inquiry, that is, for learning. Kolb (1984), Schön (1983), Bargar and Duncan (1982), and Argyris (1993) offer four models you may recognize.

David Kolb's (1984) experiential learning cycle (see Figure 3.1) is based on experiential learning theory and maps how individuals learn from experience. Kolb and Kolb describe learning as a repeating process of producing knowledge through "synergetic transactions between the person and the environment" (2005, p. 2): We have concrete experiences; we reflectively observe those experiences; we create abstract conceptualizations of those experiences; and we experiment with actions. The four activities do not necessarily occur sequentially. Ultimately, "social knowledge is created and rec- reated in the personal knowledge of the learner" (Kolb & Kolb, 2005, p. 2). The cycle illustrated in Figure 3.1.

To illustrate, we experience an event that we see, hear, touch, smell, or taste; for example, let's revisit our bread making. We remove the loaf of bread from the oven and wonder how it tastes. Eating the bread is the concrete experience. Reflective observation on the experience follows, allowing

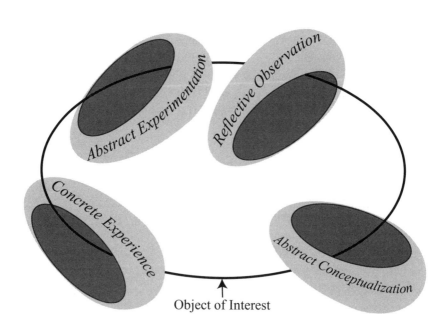

FIGURE 3.1. Kolb's learning cycle.

us to integrate the experience of the different senses and resulting in the formation of an abstract conceptualization (mmm, this bread is good). But can we be sure? So we experiment, testing with other slices of bread (maybe from the same loaf as well as others), once again having the concrete experience of tasting the bread. We are learning and relearning as we experience the bread throughout this cycle. Eventually, we decide that we prefer bread made with whole wheat flour and oatmeal and sweetened with honey.

Another practical example of an inquiry cycle is Donald Schön's (1983) reflective practice. He offers several practical illustrations in which practitioners:

- *Observe* a phenomenon;
- *Focus* on a question or surprise;
- Consciously *examine* that question;
- *Reconceptualize* the problem or puzzle; and
- *Experiment* and take action.

For example, Schön tells of the teacher who observes a child having difficulty learning to read. The teacher is puzzled because the child seems capable, so he wonders what about his own instruction is bothering the child. He asks himself: What is going on here? Because so many possible explanations exist, he has to experiment "then and there, in the classroom" (1983, p. 66), rethinking his repertoire and inventing new methods. Schön gives other examples of practitioners where "something falls outside the range of ordinary expectations" (p. 68), causing puzzlement, surprise, or confusion. Moving through the cycle, the practitioner then reflects-in-action and "becomes a researcher in the practice context" (p. 68).

Inquiry may entail confusion!

Similarly, Bargar and Duncan (1982) suggest a learning cycle that focuses on creativity as they argue for the need for creativity in doctoral research. Creative students move though the following experiences:

- *Preparation or immersion,* which includes sensing and defining a problem; building a base of information, skills, and resources; and identifying and articulating alternative perspectives (e.g., reading widely in the literature);
- *Incubation,* which may appear to be overt inactivity, where it is

presumed that the mind is sorting, integrating, synthesizing, and clarifying at a preconscious level (e.g., going for a walk, doing yoga, running);

- *Illumination* or *insight,* in which there is the emergence of an image, idea, or perspective that helps focus the problem—the "aha!" (e.g., a schematic way to organize a literature review); and

Inquiry involves insight.

- *Verification* or *development*, where developing and working through the implications of the insight take place (e.g., developing various sections of a literature review).

A more complex and challenging cycle of learning can be found in the work of Chris Argyris (1993). He posits that learning occurs when a mismatch exists between a goal, intent, or value and the consequences of action. What he calls single-loop learning results in modifying the action, whereas double-loop learning calls for a reexamination of the underlying assumptions, or "governing variables." The process is depicted in Figure 3.2.

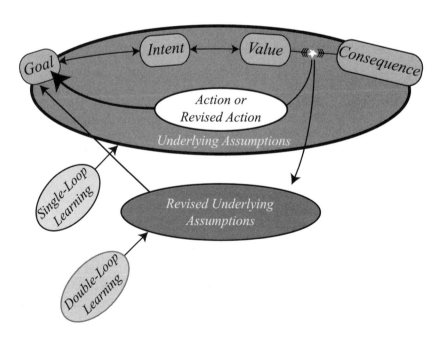

FIGURE 3.2. Argyris's learning cycle.

To illustrate, we draw on an example from research Rallis conducted in an educational setting for institutionalized youth. Every day after lunch the youth had serious difficulty settling down to the academic demands of the afternoon classes; if they were not misbehaving, they were falling asleep. At first, the faculty and staff reverted to traditional methods of control and punishment, none of which met with any success. So they began to examine their assumptions (i.e., that the youth *should* and *could* behave in class during the hour after eating lunch), only to realize that these assumptions were foolish and ungrounded in reality. All they had to do was observe the youth to see that they had lots of energy to expend after eating, so how could the adults expect them to settle down at desks to work? The faculty and staff redesigned the schedule to provide an outdoor learning activity to follow lunch. The activity allowed the youth to work off some of the energy. Surprise! The behavior problems disappeared (for the most part).

Each of these models gives insight into how people and organizations undertake the process of inquiry and learning. However, unlike the inquiring practitioner, we, as researchers, define inquiry slightly different. Whereas practitioners are free to leave their inquiry processes unexplored or as unconscious acts, researchers set out to explicate their inquiry process in an effort to legitimize and ground their work.

> Inquiry is iterative and recursive . . . never-ending.

Thus, to us, as researchers, inquiry is a planned, purposeful, and systematic process for collecting information, making decisions, and taking action as a means of contributing to knowledge generally and, more specifically, for improving policies, programs, and/or practice in order to enhance human well-being (see Weiss, 1998). With curiosity, you engage in an inquiry cycle that iteratively frames and examines problems, puzzles, or curiosities you have identified. The cycle formalizes and systematizes the natural process that humans use when making decisions. As you may notice in each of these cycles, both thinking and doing—reflection and action—are required. We have found it useful to think of inquiry as *praxis*, that is, informed action (Freire, 1970), the process of putting theoretical or abstract knowledge into action or practice.

The inquiry process is both ongoing and iterative and not necessarily linear. In practice, as we have seen, inquiry processes take various forms. Inquiry is a developing process, a cycle that builds upon itself, what Dewey calls a "reflex arc" (1896, p. 357). When Donald Schön (1983) describes reflection-on-action and reflection-in-action as producing professional knowledge, he is speaking of inquiry. The choice of specific techniques and strategies is situational, varying according to and driven by the problem at hand. *How* you choose to investigate a problem or inform a question depends on *what* the problem or question is. While inquiry is a natural and everyday human activity, scientists have staked a claim to a systematic, rigorous, and disciplined inquiry process called research. But, as we know, even babies do it.

THE SYSTEMATIC INQUIRY CYCLE

Scientists use what they call the scientific method. In a bare-bones version, scientists:

- Are curious and ask a question;
- Construct a hypothesis;
- Observe and collect data or test the hypothesis by doing an experiment;
- Analyze the data and draw a conclusion;
- Communicate results; and
- Repeat or replicate the experiment.

This method or cycle has been adopted, adapted, and applied whenever people have questions to inform or problems to solve. In professional settings, people generally follow an inquiry cycle whose activities look like Figure 3.3.

Note that the professional cycle does not refer to replication because no inquiry process in social settings can be conducted exactly as a previous one: Time has passed, people change, and circumstances will be quite different. However, the process is iterative; actions and effects are evaluated by revisiting the original problem of interest and relevant questions and by repeating the cycle under the new conditions.

Systematic inquiry then, is a process of making explicit decisions about data, about the gathering of those data, and about their meaning. What makes the cycle systematic is that it is a deliberate patterned transparent process that must be explicated so that others may understand how it was

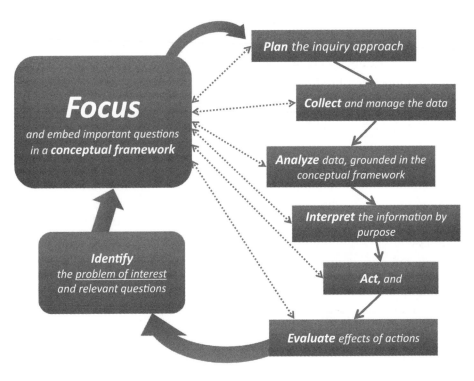

FIGURE 3.3. The cycle of inquiry.

done and can assess its adequacy and trustworthiness. The result of the process is new information or a verification or elaboration of existing information. Using this information to improve some aspect of the human condition turns it into knowledge.

Use of the cycle, which begins and ends with questions, is crucial to improving practice; it generates knowledge from which professionals can *learn* and on which they can *act*. The cycle is exactly that—not always linear and sequential. Each activity is essential for the learning, and inquiry is embedded in each activity. The cycle involves equivocal choices and interpretations that are "indeterminate, inscrutable, ambivalent, questionable, and permit multiple meanings" (Weick, 1979, p. 174). Ultimately, it is *heuristic*, a discovery process.

According to the National Research Council (NRC) (see Shavelson & Towne, 2002), research studies do the following:

- Pose *significant questions* that can be investigated empirically;
- Link research to *relevant theory*;
- Use methods that permit *direct investigation* of the questions;
- Provide a coherent and explicit *chain of reasoning*;
- Replicate and *generalize* across studies; and
- Disclose research to encourage *professional scrutiny and critique.*

However, we have found that these principles of systematic inquiry, when read and discussed in the abstract, are difficult for students to grasp. We offer several learning activities at the end of this chapter to help ground these ideas. The first activity is conducting "walk-throughs," one pedagogical strategy that we use for several aspects of the inquiry cycle. At the end of this chapter, we use it for students to practice generating and refining the topics for their projects (see Learning Activity 3.1), and we revisit it in Chapter 5 as a strategy for helping to develop the conceptual framework that guides an inquiry project.

> What is "systematic" inquiry?

In sum, scientific inquiry is a "continual process of *rigorous reasoning* supported by a dynamic interplay among methods, theories, and findings. . . . Advances in scientific knowledge are achieved by the *self-regulating norms of the scientific community* over time, not, as sometimes believed, by the mechanistic application of a particular method to a static set of questions" (Shavelson & Towne, 2002, p. 2, emphasis added). Using this definition, we see that what scientists know changes over time, as Thomas Kuhn (1962) makes clear in what he calls scientific revolutions. Indeed, "science is a social enterprise conducted by a community of inquirers operating with their own conventions . . . [where] norms and background assumptions adopted by those in the scientific community affect the course of science" (Bredo, 2006).

As you come to understand what is accepted as scientific inquiry, you see the uncertainty, the indefiniteness of knowledge. Still, the relevant scientific community must believe in the knowledge produced through systematic inquiry—that is, research; the results must stand for some acceptable version of reality. Trustworthiness, or validation, lies within what Mishler has labeled a "community of scientists" (1990, p. 422) that identifies shared definitions, as in the NRC's list presented previously, to guide their research. Rather than dismiss traditional formulations of validity that are based on experimental models as either misguided or irrelevant for social scientists, Mishler argues for a "reformulation" (p. 416) that acknowledges the social construction of knowledge (recall Berger & Luckmann, 1967). In his experience, validation is a process embedded in the social discourse among researchers; this discourse is what establishes principles and rules for any relevant domain of inquiry.

VALIDITY, CREDIBILITY, AND TRUSTWORTHINESS

"Judging the soundness and credibility of research is central to scholarship, policy development, program design, and practice. What to believe—what to put one's trust in—is foundational to the development of further research, sound policies, and programs that are designed on credible knowledge" (Rossman, Rallis, & Kuntz, 2010, p. 505). Historically, reliability, validity, objectivity, and generalizability were viewed as the standards against which to judge all research. However, these four canonical criteria have been challenged owing to multiple and sometimes conflicting assumptions about the nature of truth (what we claim we know), reality (what we claim we know about), knowledge production (how we produce those claims), and evidence (what we argue supports those claims). We discussed these multiple and conflicting assumptions in Chapter 2.

What is accepted as a standard of proof or as credible evidence now is determined within the context and purpose of the research, by the specific scientific community asking the questions and seeking the answers. However, some scientific communities focus on procedural rules to determine what credible research is. In contrast and following Phillips (2006), we look beyond procedural rules to consider how the overall argument—the truth claims—is constructed from the evidence presented and how the logic connecting the evidence to the original assertions or questions is developed. What is the underlying argument? What evidence is offered? Have the researchers presented a convincing case for the tentative conclusions put forward? Phillips argues for a wide variety of evidence in making a convincing case. "The making of a case depends on the argumentation put forward: its logic, clarity, sources of evidence, warrants connecting the evidence to the assertions, and relevance. However, what is convincing varies across time, space, and sociopolitical context" (Rossman et al., 2010, p. 506).

Put simply, the researcher develops a coherent and logical argument and uses evidence to support the argument and build trustworthiness. The type and nature of that evidence, however, ultimately rest in the researcher's conceptual framework (discussed in Chapter 5). "Research does not construct evidence—people do" (Spillane & Miele, 2007, p. 47); data become evidence when people interpret them as confirming, contradicting, or complicating the argument. Thus, the value—or acceptability—of the evidence lies in its use and its relevance to the purposes of the study. That, or on its pure logical worthiness.

Thus, the inquiry process is normative; relevant communities hold the key to credibility and usefulness of the inquiry and the knowledge it generates. Communities of practice and discourse that review and critique research—its conceptualization, design, execution, and findings—offer checks and balances to ensure that "not anything goes." Given that scientific knowledge is a social construct, what do the relevant communities of practice and discourse accept as valid, reliable, useful, or trustworthy? "The key issue becomes whether the relevant community of scientists evaluates reported findings as sufficiently trustworthy to rely on them for their own work" (Mishler, 2000, p. 120). A scientist is one who puts forward her findings *and* the reasoning that led her to those findings; other scientists then contest, modify, accept, or reject—again, stating their reasoning. The process of peer review within a discipline embodies the discourse in action.

> Knowledge is partial, incomplete, and context bound.

An example from a nonacademic community of practice might help illustrate the normative nature of the inquiry process. The medical profession uses grand rounds as both a diagnostic and a teaching tool. Grand rounds are formal lectures during which physicians, residents, medical students, and other medical personnel discuss each patient's clinical case. The medical problems and treatment of a particular patient are described, questioned, and critiqued to document the patient's progress, evaluate treatment, and propose alternatives. These rounds follow a prescribed heuristic ritual so that participants know what to expect and how they may contribute; the ritual results in teaching new information, developing clinical reasoning skills, and generating knowledge—it is inquiry in action.

But, we ask, what about the patient? Shouldn't he have a say in what knowledge ensues? If other scientists are the only source of validation claims, won't all knowledge validation be accomplished through a privileged and potentially biased lens? What about practitioners and others who may use what scientists produce? Should not usefulness be a criterion for the validity as well as value of any research? We suggest that the normative group, especially in social sciences whose aim is to produce knowledge to serve the human population, often extends—and should extend—beyond scientists. Just as Mishler (1990) notes the presence of conflict and controversy in science, we note that the principles and rules morph as multiple voices enter, fueling conflict and controversy to transform the dialogue. Thus, the dialogue must be inclusive as well as continuous, ongoing, and ever changing— a form of democratic deliberation.

With its recursiveness, inquiry enacts the indefiniteness of knowledge. That is, as inquiry guides further exploration and reevaluation, it mirrors the changing nature of truth and growing diversity of understanding. It is, as Dewey posits, context bound and self-correcting. Inquiry is, in essence, shared; it sits within a community as we put forward our process to others. Knowing suggests a particular *normative status*. No claim to knowledge can be determined apart from connection with a widening circle of consequences. "Inquiry in a given special field appeals to the experiences of the community of fellow workers for confirmation and correction of his results" (Dewey, 1938, p. 56). An answer or solution that "does not fit or function well necessitates some transformation of the inquiry" (Johnston, 2006, p. 60); in other words, research that cannot meet professional scrutiny and critique is either discredited, ignored, or modified to meet the acceptable standards.

Education professionals' views toward educating persons with disabilities illustrate the emergent nature of what is considered valid as knowledge. When we began teaching, children with disabilities were considered handicapped and placed in special settings, if educated at all. Research on the brain, multiple intelligences, and learning disabilities offered new knowledge about how people learn and how various disabilities interact with learning. Previously held "truths" were challenged and called into question. Public interest groups entered the conversation, adding experience and passion—and advocacy. A reformulated understanding of what disability is and its place in education resulted. A deliberation among scientists and the public defined—is still defining—validity in our knowledge of disabilities.

Recognizing that knowledge production requires professional scrutiny demonstrates the dialogical nature of all inquiry. The notion of dialogical interchange is, literally, a back-and-forth process, as illustrated in

> Knowledge claims demand scrutiny by the community of practice.

the dialogue that began this chapter. In such a process, an idea is batted around and thereby not only explored but also "impacted" by each participant (or vantage point/question/personality). Much like a rock that is changed by the action of the waves on the beach, arguments and their logics are smoothed by community discourse or cracked into bits at points of inner weakness.

Dialogical interchanges have the specific aim of learning; they explore underlying meaning and assumptions for the purpose of reaching a new level of understanding. You engage in personal individual dialogue when you reason and argue with yourself. When you bring your reasoning and arguments to your classmates, you engage in dialogue with your *community of practice* (Lave & Wenger, 1991), that is, a group that meets face to face, shares common sociocultural practices, and strives toward common goals. The dialogue continues when you put forward your work to your *community of discourse*, or scholars (Nystrand, 1982); that is, you present at your professional association or you publish.

The community of practice is your peers and professors: You engage in face-to-face (or e-mail) critical discussions with them as you move through the odyssey of crafting a solid approach to your inquiry project. This process, specifically focusing on early conceptualizations of inquiry projects, was depicted in the dialogue that opened this chapter. We provide specifics to guide the critical inquiry process at the end of this chapter (see Learning Activity 3.2).

As a graduate student engaging in research and producing your own knowledge, you will, more or less, use the criteria for trustworthiness discussed previously to guide your process. As we have been saying all along, what we claim to know is a result of a complicated interaction between the knower, the known, and the context or social world. The elements of an inquiry cycle operate within this interaction and draw on the values and norms of the referent community. The inquiry cycle connects theory and practice, thinking and doing. To be trustworthy and to produce knowledge—that is, information that is used to improve the human condition—the inquiry, whether scientific, systematic, personal, or informal, must be conducted ethically. "Bad science makes for bad ethics" (Rosenthal, 1994, p. 128), and we add that bad ethics makes for bad science. The next chapter explores definitions of ethical inquiry practice.

Learning Activity 3.1. Critical Inquiry Triads

In our classes, we use the inquiry triad as a pedagogical strategy to build the critical conversations necessary for a true community of practice. Whether you use the triad as a part of a class or informally outside of class, the dialogue among the members can be invaluable for moving your ideas forward. Find a group of three (but no more) colleagues to work together on various structured or assigned tasks over the semester. Some such tasks are depicted in the dialogues at the beginnings of the chapters. Think of these inquiry triads as creating opportunities for dialogue to help you clarify and deepen your work. Partners serve as "critical friends" (Rallis & Rossman, 2000), that is, peers whose observations, feedback, and critical (but gentle) questions enhance learning. As a corollary benefit, these dialogues have proven valuable for each member of the triad.

For the inquiry triad, we ask: What does *critical* mean? In surfacing various conceptions, we stress that the term implies critique, not criticism. Critique relies on both positive and negative feedback for the purpose of improving the work at hand. Critical also means "essential"; essential questions explore the heart of the issues and recognize the tentative and speculative nature of any answers.

We further elaborate that critical inquiry aims to explore *alternative perspectives* and, therefore, demands open-mindedness on the part of the receiver of the question. Considering alternatives is crucial for building intriguing, robust conceptual frameworks and generative inquiry designs. Think back to the Learning Activity 2.2: Alternative Maps. Critical questions are often grounded in a social justice framework and seek to discover a more just system. A typical social justice question asks, "Whose interests are or are not being served by this perspective?"

Critical inquiry also seeks *change*. Derived from the concept of critical mass in physics, similar to Piaget's (1953) assertion of the centrality of disequilibrium for learning, and captured in the widely popular book *The Tipping Point* (Gladwell, 2000), critical inquiry at best fosters a reconceptualization of the topic and thus new insights and potential approaches. Critical inquiry triad partners move from equilibrium ("I'm sure I know what's going on here") through disequilibrium ("Um, perhaps there are other ways to view this?") to a new understanding ("That's how I'll approach it, but I need to remain open") that is grounded but open to modification.

Necessary Conditions

- *Purpose and material*—you have to have something to talk about;
- *Trust* that comes from mutual benefit—you learn from helping one another;
- *A risk-encouraging* environment—no final judgments; and
- *A willingness to search out* and listen to other voices.

Tips and Skills

1. Ask questions:
   - To clarify: What do you mean by . . .?
   - To establish purpose and consequence: What might happen if . . .?
   - To identify alternative perspectives: Had you considered . . .?
   - To link ideas and observations to other experiences and theories: How does this connect to . . .?
   - To extend ideas: What if you thought about . . .?
2. Help your partners establish focus.
3. Base the dialogue on your partners' work.
4. Be sure you understand and probe for deeper understanding (no question is too basic); share your impressions and observations.
5. Keep in mind the goal of helping your partners explore answers to their questions.

This pedagogical strategy is quite useful in helping to build a community of practice among your colleagues that is crucial for developing inquiry-mindedness. Such communities prove valuable for developing logical, credible, and interesting conceptual frameworks and, ultimately, research proposals. Central is the notion of building a convincing argument, which is facilitated by identifying and making transparent your interests in as well as potential biases regarding the topic.

Learning Activity 3.2. "Walk-Throughs" to Find a Problem, Question, or Surprise

In many of our research classes, we use an activity called a _walk-through_. The activity is sufficiently open to serve many purposes; here, we discuss how it is used in helping to locate and perhaps refine a possible topic.

A walk-through is an activity in which one person volunteers to informally present his potential inquiry topic to the entire class, or if your class or group is large (more than 12), to smaller groups of about six. You could even use your _Critical Inquiry Triad_, described in the previous activity. The volunteer begins by talking about the topic and how he became interested in it (personal or professional interest). Give the volunteer 5–10 minutes to talk, without questions or comments from the others.

Then open up the discussion, reminding your group members that clarifying questions or comments are most appropriate at this point. You might review the guidelines for brainstorming: that any comment is potentially useful; that the purpose is to broaden the volunteer's thinking; that the volunteer does not need to respond to a specific question, but merely consider it. Ask someone to serve as "scribe," writing comments and questions on the chalkboard or flip-chart paper. When group members have made comments or posed questions for about 20 minutes, it becomes the volunteer's time to respond and share with the class how the comments may (or may not) help him narrow down his topic.

We have found that walk-throughs are quite useful for illuminating the challenges involved in focusing an inquiry project. The volunteer's concrete example makes this process come alive and vividly demonstrates the iterative, often messy, process of defining and refining a topic. During the walk-throughs, materials you may have presented earlier often become clearer. A primary purpose here is to explore decisions involved in conceptualizing and designing solid research.

FOR FURTHER READING

Argyris, C. (1993). _On organizational learning_. Cambridge, MA: Blackwell.

Burke, P. J. (2009). _The elements of inquiry: A guide for consumers and producers of research_. Glendale, CA: Pyrczak.

Dewey, J. (1938). _Logic: The theory of inquiry_. New York: Holt.

➥ Getzels, J. W. (1982). The problem of the problem. In R. M. Hogarth (Ed.), *Question framing and response consistency* (pp. 37–49). San Francisco: Jossey-Bass.

➥ Kolb, D. A. (1984). *Experiential learning: Experience as the source of learning and development*. Englewood Cliffs, NJ: Prentice Hall.

➥ Lundberg, C. C., & Young, C. A. (Eds.). (2005). *Foundations for inquiry: Choices and trade-offs in the organizational sciences*. Stanford, CA: Stanford Business Books.

➥ Schön, D. A. (1983). *The reflective practitioner: How professionals think in action*. New York: Basic Books.

CHAPTER 4

Being an Ethical Inquirer
Staying Alert on the Road

⊛ *Critical Questions to Guide Your Reading*

⇀ *What ethical considerations do I need to be aware of? (remembering)* Power - representation, respect, justice

⇀ *In what ways do universities, funding agencies, and associations monitor ethics? (understanding)*

⇀ *What are major ethical theories? (remembering)*

⇀ *How do these theories differ from one another? (analyzing)*

⇀ *Why does reasoning and reflecting about issues that come up help ensure a trustworthy study? (analyzing)*

⇀ *How do I anticipate or forecast what benefits there might be for participants? What about potential harm to them? (applying)*

⇀ *How will I know I've made an ethical choice? (evaluating)*

Dialogue 4. What Ethical Considerations Might Affect My Project?

As the students in Bettara's class move forward—in fits and starts—with thinking about inquiry generally and their own projects specifically, the professor asked them to share their ideas about ethical research practice. They are stumped, because they aren't sure what ethical practice is. Their dialogue:

KEVIN: I've got an idea. Remember the reading on principals doing action research in their own schools? Well, some of those ideas struck me pretty hard. Especially the idea that I'm "the boss." What do you think about that? Does it matter?

SAMIRA: Hmm. But those authors said it was OK to do that kind of research. And haven't we read about other situations like that? When there are all sorts of power stuff in the setting?

REILLY: This is my turf! There're all sorts of power in universities, especially power over students. Obviously, researchers also play with power. I read something about how deception is OK in research because we all do it anyway—something about "managing impressions."

MARTINA: Can we get back to Kevin's point? It's different from yours, Reilly. Kevin is asking about when we—the researchers—have some sort of power over the folks in the study. That's different, I think.

SAMIRA: You guys know that I'm interested in social justice issues—we say that fairness and equity supercede other interests. I guess a power lens would ask who defines what is fair and equitable. And we argue that everything is influenced by the power hierarchies; people just don't recognize them. So, is it different for you, Kevin?

KEVIN: Well, I'm not sure. I have a great relationship with the teachers . . . At least *I* think I do—maybe they see it differently! Anyway, for my study, I won't be "evaluating" them; I'll just learn more about what they are doing that seems to work for these boys. Doesn't my purpose fall under that "beneficence" category? And that makes it OK, doesn't it?

RAUL: Look. The deal here is that Kevin *does* evaluate the teachers—midyear, at the end of the year. He writes recommendations for them. He's got a lot of power, even though we all know that he's a nice guy. Kevin, those teachers know about that power, and it affects how they act toward you. That makes it pretty complicated. I mean, they might fear you'll use their answers to judge the way they deal with boys.

SAMIRA: Can we tie this conversation to ethical research practice? Are we even certain what "ethics" is? I mean, ethics is not only about power, is it? It's about respect too, isn't it? I think it comes down to how Kevin talks with them and how he writes about what he learns.

REILLY: It's not just about Kevin's position or intent, Samira. As you just said, one of the things that matters is how he writes about them. Remember that reading we did? The prof from Alabama who studied faculty? He had lots of troubles because those faculty members were concerned about how he "represented" them. Remember? The article in QSE?

MARTINA: Yes, I recall that one. He was a student in Bettara's class about 5 years ago! So his issues were all about telling too much about the faculty—they were real concerned that he was only going to tell his own perspective. He was worried about that respect issue Samira mentioned. Does anyone remember what he did?

RAUL: Sure, I do. He wrote memos . . . a whole lot of them! Mostly to himself, as I recall. But also to his chair. I think that helped him get more clear about what to do.

MARTINA: But I'm still not sure what his ethical decisions were. I still need to know more about how we can use the readings to think through what we're going to do in our own studies.

RAUL: Right. But even if we think it through now, stuff is still going to come up—stuff we can't imagine right now.

The students continue grappling with the issues of power and representation, respect and justice, trying to surface the deep concerns that underlie specific research projects. As this dialogue unfolds, they engage with the everyday issues that arise for an ethical research practitioner.

ETHICS IN INQUIRY

As we said in Chapter 3, trustworthiness is foundational to conducting inquiry that will produce credible and useful knowledge. We also argue that inquiry, as a value-laden enterprise, demands ethical practice. But first, like Samira, you may be wondering exactly what "ethics" is and what ethics has

> Beneficence, respect for persons, justice = your anchors.

to do with inquiry. We define ethics as *standards for conduct that are based on moral principles*. As a researcher, your moral principles—what you consider to be good or bad, right or wrong—define your ethics and thus, your character, which guides your actions. Put simply, moral principles provide the rules that offer guidance for how you act in any given situation. Thus, ethical research practice is guided by moral principles, and with our claim that all research should have a goal of improving some aspect of the human condition, we establish a moral position. We now move to a discussion of the ethics of inquiry.

Because the inquiry cycle models presented in the last chapter may imply a step-by-step approach to generating knowledge, we are concerned that you might assume that ethical research practice also follows step-by-step procedures. Such is *not* the case. In fact, over the past several years, our work (Rallis, 2006a, 2006b, 2010; Rallis & Rossman, 2003, 2004, 2010; Rallis, Rossman, & Gajda, 2007; Rossman & Rallis, 1998, 2003, 2010, 2012[2]) has critiqued the dominance of procedures—the step-by-step approaches required by university regulations—over moral principles to guide the ethics of research practice. During our years of practice as academics, researchers, and supervisors of dissertation research, we have seen attention to procedural matters overtake the bedrock principles of respect for persons, beneficence, and justice that are encoded in institutional policies for the protection of human subjects in research. We have found that the public discourse—in university hallways and classrooms—focuses on getting the procedural matters right rather than on getting the ethical matters right. In fact, seldom does the discourse even recognize ethics. However, because most of the research being conducted around us (whether in, for example, education, public policy, public health, management, or psychology) involves humans, we are concerned with how researchers relate to the persons who participate in studies. Deep engagement with people means that ethical matters will arise in the everyday conduct of research.

The everyday ethical issues that arise—Kevin's and those of the author of the study on university professors mentioned in the opening dialogue (see Kuntz, 2010)—are moments that demand moral considerations and ethical choices. "The point of moral principles is to regulate interactions among human beings" (Strike, Haller, & Soltis, 1998, p. 41). Moral reasoning and its corollary sensibilities should, we argue, become part of a researcher's daily practice. We begin by introducing the researcher as a

---

[2] Much of this chapter draws on this body of work.

moral practitioner. We then turn to concerns raised within communities of discourse about the tendency to observe merely obligatory ethical procedures as outlined in human subjects review regulations and frequently encoded in the iconic informed consent letter. Because, in our view, these procedural rituals are grossly inadequate for the moral challenges of research with people, we invite you to engage deeply with the ethical dilemmas and defining moments that may well arise in the everyday conduct of research. To inform this engagement, we present various theories of ethics. However, because theories are necessarily abstract, we end this chapter with practical considerations.

THE INQUIRER AS A MORAL PRACTITIONER

Recall that we see inquiry as a kind of *praxis*—the ebb and flow of thinking and doing, theorizing and gathering data, writing and reflecting. These ideas are all embedded in the inquiry cycle models presented in Chapter 3. If inquiry is a kind of praxis, then we can see that the inquirer is a *practitioner* and, we hope, a reflective one, as Schön would have it. Practitioners are decision makers; they follow a chain of reasoning in which moral principles are integral. Every decision about data collection, analysis, interpretation, and presentation has moral dimensions. Thus, their decisions cover both the procedural and ethical matters that attend the conduct of research, especially when the research is focused on human well-being (Hostetler, 2005).

> What is your inquiry practice?

As the dialogue that begins this chapter depicts, these decisions are ongoing and demand iterative reflection and action. Ethical researchers will encounter moments and situations that demand moral consideration. Thus, researchers might rightly be considered to be *moral practitioners* (see Sikes & Goodson, 2003). Morally compelling moments demand a reflexivity that we call *research praxis*—that is, informed action, the back-and-forth between reasoning and action. Methodological wisdom emerges during the cyclical process of inquiry that is doing, thinking about the doing through a moral lens, and doing again. We hope that, as you begin your inquiry journeys, you take quite seriously the notion that morally grounded researchers are ethically reflexive practitioners.

> Strive to become a moral practitioner of inquiry.

As a practitioner, a researcher who engages in systematic inquiry continually makes decisions about design and data collection, analysis, interpretation, and reporting. What makes the inquiry systematic and scholarly is transparency, that is, the willingness and ability of the researcher to put forward her reasoning for critique within both the community of practice and the relevant community of scholars. We argue that because each decision has an effect on the study's participants and the relationship between them and the researcher, each decision is ethical and thus demands moral consideration. An ethical researcher, then, is bound to articulate the moral bases for her inquiry decisions. We suggest that doing so has the added benefit of making explicit the study's purpose, logic, and potential expectations of and benefits to the participants, thus foreshadowing possible ethical questions.

Such decisions, while grounded in the conceptual framework of the inquiry project or research study, continue to be developed and modified as the research becomes practice. The practitioner "is *in* the situation that he seeks to understand," is "in conversation with it" (Schön, 1983, p. 151); the phenomenon influences the practitioner, and he influences the phenomenon. The inquirer's relation to the situation is a dynamic interaction. Schön (1983) describes the process as a hypothesis-testing experiment or game:

> [The inquirer's] activity is neither self-fulfilling prophecy, nor is it the neutral hypothesis testing of the method of the controlled experiment. The *practice situation* is neither clay to be molded at will nor an independent, self-sufficient object of study from which the inquirer keeps his distance. (p. 150, emphasis added)

In short, an ethical researcher does more than reflect; he *reflects-in-action*. At the same time that the inquirer tries to understand the situation within the study's frame, "he holds himself open to the situation's back talk" (Schön, 1983, p. 164). We call this simultaneous awareness of the self and other, and of the interplay between the two, *reflexive practice* "in the sense that it provides us with ways of talking about research on practice that treats research itself as practice. We need to find ways of turning our approach to research back on itself so that it becomes critically recursive" (Schratz & Walker, 1995, p. 13).

Recognizing research as reflexive practice foregrounds the relational matters; doing so moves considerations of trustworthiness beyond merely technical or procedural matters. Moreover, because reflexive practice defines the ultimate outcome of research as knowledge—that is, information that may contribute to the improvement of the human condition—the moral imperative is strengthened. Every decision considers both consequential (the outcome) and nonconsequential (the process) ethical theories. Thus, ethical and competent researchers exercise probity; that is, they reason through moral principles with integrity.

STANDARDS FOR PRACTICE
AND PROCEDURAL MATTERS

Standards for ethical research practice are found in federal regulations, funding agencies, professional associations, and licensure boards, among others. Ethical inquirers are aware of these and pay attention to their codes and norms. In decades past, numerous instances of unethical research (see, e.g., Punch, 1994, for descriptions) led the U.S. government and professional associations to set standards and, in some cases, to intervene in order to protect human subjects. The federal government has established clear standards for researchers in any institution or organization that receives federal funds; they must comply with regulations that define ethical practice. At universities, questions about how researchers relate to their participants—the ethical matters—have fallen under the jurisdiction of institutional review boards (IRBs). These boards, a familiar function at most universities, have the responsibility to ensure the protection of human subjects in all the research conducted under the auspices of that institution. IRBs serve important roles because they judge what is considered ethical practice with human subjects. Individual autonomy, privacy, and harm form the foundation of the framework behind the three ethical principles guiding IRB deliberations (originally stipulated in *The Belmont Report*; National Commission for the Protection of Human Subjects of Biomedical and Behavioral Research, 1979): Respect for Persons, Beneficence, and Justice. *Respect for Persons* means that researchers are to treat subjects as independent agents; those who cannot act independently are considered vulnerable and must be protected. *Beneficence* considers the researchers' obligation to maximize possible benefits and minimize potential harms. *Justice* refers to the balance of who receives benefits from the research and who bears its burdens (Hemmings, 2006, provides a more complete discussion). IRBs have applied the principles through a requirement

Procedures or principles?

that informed consent must be secured from participants; this consent affirms the subject's understanding of the research purposes, benefits, and possible harms, and states how the researchers will guarantee the subject's privacy (confidentiality and anonymity).

IRBs and their institutions usually require researchers to receive certification from the Collaborative Institutional Training Initiative (*www. citiprogram.org/citidocuments/aboutus.htm*). Although the modules in this training are quite informative and interesting, they are insufficient to ensure that on-the-ground research conduct is truly ethical. In fact, IRBs often require a set of procedures that simplifies the incredibly complex ethical issues that arise. Thus, we argue that approval by this board is hardly sufficient. We support the claim that "there is no direct or necessary relationship between ethics committee approval of a research project and what actually happens when the research is undertaken" (Guillemin & Gillam, 2004, p. 269). Within the research relationship, practical tensions are present: harm and burden versus respect and benefit. Avoiding harm (physical, emotional, or social) is basic (Guillemin & Gillam, 2004), and bearing undue burden may be harmful (see Hemmings, 2006). However, in all research, potentials for harm "are often quite subtle and stem from the nature of the interaction between researcher and participant" (Guillemin & Gillam, 2004, p. 272). Similarly, forecasting potential benefits to participation in a research study is sometimes tricky, as the researchers may anticipate benefits that then do not accrue. Yet the IRB, through its emblematic letter of informed consent, has come to serve as one of the primary formal gatekeepers to ethical practice. As noted, professional associations and research foundations also serve as ethics gatekeepers, because both have standards for ethical research practice (see, e.g., the American Evaluation Association's Guiding Principles for Evaluators, available at *www.eval.org/publications/guiding-principles.asp*). We list a few other associations' codes of ethics at the end of this chapter.

To illustrate, let's look more closely at the letter of consent. Obtaining a person's signature on a letter of consent is, at minimum, a contract. It serves as a proxy indicator of the participant's trust in the researcher: *I trust that you will respect my rights and needs; I trust that you will protect me from harm; I trust that your selection of me as a participant is just and that there are benefits to me for participating (not just you).* Establishing trust requires more than a contract; it requires interactions grounded in the three principles described previously. But, in any specific research context, what constitutes respect, beneficence, and justice? Only the researcher and the participants, dialoging together, can say how these principles play out in practice.

The dialogue recognizes the individuality of the participants in the specific context of the study: Who are these people? Why have they been chosen, and why have they agreed to participate? Do they truly understand what you expect of them? Can they agree voluntarily without pressure or obligation? What are the likely benefits to them for participating? Participants may hold very different views of the study's purposes and the concept of voluntary consent. Certainly, characteristics such as age, cultural background, position, and level of education influence participants' understanding and expectations. For many studies, researchers decide to write letters in a language that participants can understand, whether that language is Spanish, Urdu, at a child's level, geared to parents, and so on. Other times, they may decide a signature is inappropriate. Often, researchers have to think on their feet when talking with participants about informed consent. Next, we offer two scenarios that presented surprises and required far more than a simple signature[3]:

> **Setting the scene:** A small southern African nation that is trying desperately to implement Education for All but has recently enacted policies that prevent students from maximizing their chances to be selected to secondary school. In this setting, selection to secondary school represents a life-changing opportunity. Therefore, policies that indirectly or inadvertently constrain those chances have a profoundly negative effect on the development of the nation's human resources. Because the design calls for interviews of secondary school personnel in an effort to understand how these policies impact selected villages, the researcher presents the study participants with an informed consent letter.
>
> **R:** I thank you for your willingness to be interviewed. As you know, we want to learn how you operate under the various policies related to students' selection for secondary schools. First, I need to have you sign this piece of paper that will give your consent to be interviewed—it is called an informed consent letter. It simply describes the study that I have told you about and promises that I will protect your privacy. I'll record your answers, but nobody else will hear the tape and I will not use your name in the report.

---

[3] See Rallis et al. (2007) for a more thorough description and discussion of these cases.

P: Who sent you here? The government?

R: No, an NGO [nongovernmental organization] has funded the study—we want to understand the selection process for secondary school: What helps students be selected? What stands in the way of their being selected? How do the policies affect who are your students and how you work with them?

P: Why did you choose me? Have I done anything wrong?

R: No—not at all! I want to talk with you because you teach in a secondary school so you live with the results of the selection process.

P: I would like to talk with you about the problems that stand in the way of our students entering secondary schooling. I am pleased you are interested. But I am sorry. I will not sign any form.

R: The form is essential—I cannot interview unless you sign it. It ensures that you understand the study and that you agree.

P: No, if I sign, I will be on a list. That is dangerous.

R: I won't be keeping any list. I will store the letter in a secure file, but I'll be sure your name does not appear on any papers.

P: The only times we are asked to sign is when there is a problem with the government. How can I know that won't happen with this piece of paper?

R: Maybe we should talk more about what I will be doing in the study—and why I am doing the study. I am hoping the results can be helpful to you, can help modify policies that impede and support those that facilitate access to secondary schools.

P: Please do tell me more—I want to understand how the study can help us. And I do want to talk with you. But I will not sign a paper.

Setting the scene: In a large urban U.S. city, a group of women who have survived physical abuse have banded together and secured funding to provide counseling and support groups for women in shelters who are escaping abusive relationships. The funder wants to know what services have been provided and how they have been used, and so has sent an evaluator to interview a sample of women who have received the services and participated in the groups.

E: I appreciate your taking the time to talk with me. As you know, the Setag Foundation has made possible the *Roofless Women* Project.

They are interested in what your participation has meant to you. I'd like to ask you to tell me what you have done with *Roofless Women*—and whether you think the counselors and meeting with other women like yourself has helped you. But before we begin, I need to ask you to sign this paper. We call it an informed consent letter—it describes the project and what I will do with your interview. Your signature indicates that you understand the study and that you agree.

P: I'm a little nervous about talking with you. I mean, what if I say the wrong things?

E: There are no "wrong things." I mean, what we want is to know what you think about *Roofless Women*.

P: Who is going to hear this?

E: Actually, no one will hear the tape but me and the transcriber—someone who will not know who you are. Your name won't be on the interview—and then I'll erase the tape.

P: And who will read the report? Are they people who can hurt us?

E: To the contrary—I'm hoping that what we learn can help to improve the services you are receiving. Possibly bring more support for services for you and others.

P: I don't know. Some things aren't that good, so I might say something someone does not like. What if someone figures out it is me? I mean, there are not so many of us. And what will you do with what I say, even if you don't put my name on it.

E: Tell me why this bothers you so much?

P: Well, I mean, this is pretty personal. I would not want certain people to see what I say. How do I know I can trust you?

E: I see what you mean—and I certainly respect your feelings. Even if you sign it you can always opt out at any point—it says so in the letter. If you sign it, we can just begin talking about your experience with *Roofless Women*, and you can see how you feel about our conversation. If you are not comfortable, you can just stop. The only point of the letter is to ensure that you know you are doing this because you want to, without pressure.

P: Well, maybe, but why am I one of the people you are talking to? Am I so screwed up that you want to see how much trouble I'm in?

E: You may see yourself that way but I do not know anything like that about you. All I know is that you have lived at the shelter and joined *Roofless Women*.

P: But why did you choose me?

E: Well, I'd guess you have a story to tell—and you can help me get that story to the funders so they can decide if the program is worthwhile. And you are a person who could benefit from improved services.

P: Do you mean this program might not continue?

E: I'm not saying that but the foundation did ask me to give them information on the value of the program. Whatever you can tell me might help them to decide if they should continue to support the program or maybe improve the services.

P: But what if I say something bad about the counselor? What if I say we need more money?

E: I'll present those issues as possible problems with the service delivery—I won't identify you as the person who said it. Besides, there may be others who feel the way you do. The program people may choose to change things you and others point out.

P: Hmm, so—are you saying that they might listen to me?

E: I cannot guarantee what the program people will do. I will tell you that I will communicate to those in charge what I learn from the women I talk with. My purpose is to see that the services are beneficial and improved if they need to be.

P: I still don't know if I should trust you. How do I know you won't change my words?

E: What I can do is show you the transcript from the tape. You can see if there are mistakes. I admit I am the one who interprets what you say.

P: What do you mean by that?

E: As I read what you and the other women say, I figure out what is the message to send to the foundation and the program people. I guess you have to trust me—or the group of you can work with me. We can talk about what the major issues are and how to say them to the funders. So, do you want to go ahead with the interview?

P: Yeah, I guess so. I'll sign that paper—but, you know, I may decide to stop.

E: I agree, you can do that. Let's see how it goes.

These scenarios illustrate collaborative dialogues that establish shared definitions and begin to build a level of trust between the researchers and their participants. Without collaborative dialogue to establish expectations and conditions, a signature on a consent letter becomes merely a procedural way to *attempt to* ensure ethical behavior and establish trust. Instead, "informed consent is a respectful communication process, not a consent form" and wise researchers modify and even radically alter procedures of informed consent (Seiber, 2004, p. 496) in order to establish, develop, and preserve relationships with research participants by addressing ambiguities and creating shared understandings.

As we have witnessed over the years, this proceduralization of ethics has had important consequences: Graduate students often speak in coded language about IRB approval, appearing to believe that such approval certifies their research as "ethical"; investigators assume that approval means they can proceed without further consideration of rights, justice, or beneficence; participants unconsciously trust that the researchers will honor the relationship. Sample informed consent letters are a standard requirement of a review board's procedures. Obtaining informed consent from participants—and the forms that guide this—seems to have become more important than true ethical engagement. This, to us, represents a troubling codification and bureaucratization of moral reasoning and ethical practice.

Sometimes we worry that sorting out the thorny issues associated with ongoing ethical practice becomes tedious and unproductive. Moreover, cultural differences in interpretation of informed consent forms are hardly present in IRB procedures, and discussions about how to ethically write up—represent—the data are elided. Our position should be clear: Attending merely to procedures, at the cost of fully engaging with the ethical and relational matters of research with people, represents a facile misapplication of the "technical compendia that masquerade as methodology" (Nixon & Sikes, 2003, p. 5), as applied to ethical research practice. We encourage all researchers to prioritize the three principles of respect, protection from harm, and balancing burden with benefit.

ETHICS, TRUSTWORTHINESS, AND RIGOR[4]

For research to be credible, we must trust in it. This assertion is a truism but one that remains mysterious in methodological writings. Just what is

[4]This section is adapted from Rallis, Rossman, Cobb, Reagan, and Kuntz (2008) and from Rallis et al. (2007). Copyright 2008 by Corwin Press and 2007 by Elsevier Science, Ltd. Adapted by permission.

meant by trust? Trust in what? Trust in whom? And what does the derived term *trustworthiness* mean? Judgments about the trustworthiness of a study are typically made according to the normative rules and standards of a particular discipline, often relying on *procedural rules* as criteria, as introduced in Chapter 3. Traditionally, these rules have stipulated the procedures to follow to ensure the reliability, validity, objectivity, and generalizability of a study. These canons imply that the extent to which one can trust in the soundness of a study depends on whether appropriate procedures were followed—the technical matters. Was the sample size appropriate? Was the researcher objective? Was the instrumentation reliable? Were the data gathered appropriately? Notably absent are considerations of the principles and practice of ethical research. Such discussions occur separately from discussions about the canonical four. Moreover, the paramount principles of respect for human beings, beneficence, and justice are often reduced to the procedural matters of gaining informed consent, as we have noted previously. Nixon and Sikes (2003) argue that "methodology is centrally concerned with method. But method cannot be reduced to technique. Method rules, and is ruled by, the myriad adjustments, accommodations and resistances that constitute our being together" (p. 5). Put simply, procedures provide a false security. The novice researcher (and, unfortunately, the more experienced one) who relies solely on procedures is likely to produce an impoverished study.

We know of a student in psychology who was a research assistant (RA) on a study measuring the effects of an intervention with adolescents who abused alcohol. Because the study was conducted in a research university, IRB approval was required. As the RA, the student was charged with completing the varied and numerous forms that included guarantees of confidentiality and protection from harm. The required procedures were extensive and thorough; the RA fully complied, and the study received approval. Very quickly, the study ran into problems with recruitment. The participants were minors, so parental consent was required, but many potential participants did not want to reveal their alcohol use to their parents. Because the number of participants was not high enough to meet the design projections, the principal investigator (PI) demanded more effort to bring in participants and even recommended that the criteria for selection (e.g., participants had to be under a certain weight, could not be hard-drug users, could not report being depressed) be relaxed. The RA wondered how he could increase participation while still ensuring that all would be protected from possible harm. The RA also was disturbed when he heard secretaries at lunch talking about a participant and again when he witnessed a list of those who had not been selected being passed to another study; he considered these actions to be violations of the promised confidentiality. As the weeks passed, the RA began to realize that many of his efforts to comply with the IRB procedures had little connection to reality. Moreover, he realized that what he considered to be ethical violations also compromised the study: How could they claim findings were valid and reliable if participants did not even meet the study criteria?

As another example, the team of evaluators contracted to assess an ambitious citizen-driven change initiative came head to head with thorny ethical issues when dealing with consultants. To set the scene, the initiative, Podemos Hacerlo, had the goal of fostering agency—self-efficacy—among ordinary citizens such that they would feel empowered to advocate with government officials about their access to and the quality of basic services. The initiative was quite bold in scope and drew on partnerships with various organizations and networks across five countries for implementation.

The evaluation design called for gathering substantial baseline data against which to measure change, a common practice with great merit. The baseline study had two primary components: (1) nationally representative, randomly sampled surveys in the five countries targeted by the initiative and (2) a set of ethnographic case studies to gather in-depth information. In designing the baseline survey questionnaires, the sponsor, Podemos for short, suggested that the evaluation team draw on the expertise of a group of consultants who were working on measuring empowerment in various cultural contexts. The team agreed, and a process of e-mail development of survey questions ensued.

> How might participants be put at risk or harmed?

After a few months, a face-to-face workshop was planned. The evaluation team and the consultants all brought sets of questions for review, comment, and critical appraisal before preliminary field testing. Given their well-developed theoretical perspective, the consultants brought very specific questions that, they argued, were crucial for measuring empowerment. The evaluation team also brought sets of questions. Both sets were to be asked of "ordinary citizens"—*campesinos*—in the five countries.

One member of the evaluation team came from a village in a very rural area in the country where the workshop was held, and he spoke the local language where field testing was planned. His cultural sensitivities and linguistic knowledge were crucial for developing questions that would be meaningful and appropriate for campesinos. However, he felt that many of the consultants' questions were meaningless to campesinos—they assumed an individualistic social organization; they assumed an orientation to change and the future that was highly problematic in that context. He argued quite eloquently that these questions be changed prior to field testing. However, his expertise, local knowledge, and critical wisdom were ignored by the consultants. The evaluation team was deeply concerned that the ethical principle of Respect for Persons was going to be seriously compromised if the existing questions went forward.

Despite the evaluation team's best efforts, preliminary field testing of the questionnaire (a common and crucially important practice in question-naire development), including the problematic questions, was scheduled to take place in a rural town and its surrounding villages, not far from the capital city. As the team predicted, the campesinos found questions such as "When do you feel most like yourself?" and "What would you like to change in your life?" baffling and, in some cases, insulting. Their worst fears were confirmed: Many of the questions made the campesinos feel inadequate and frustrated (because they didn't know how to respond!), and the intrusion into their lives was handled with a lack of cultural and linguistic sensitivity. The evaluation team tried to soften and modify questions to better suit the real people they were interviewing, with some success. However, the team left this exercise with a deep concern about how seriously the consultants understood the deeply relational ethical matters at play. To their credit, they were open to learning how better to phrase questions, but their theoreti-cal framework meant that some of the strange and confounding questions would just have to be asked.

An example where Rallis evaluated an ethnographic study documenting qualities of innovative schools illustrates how even experienced researchers can ignore relationships and defer only to procedures. The PI was a senior researcher with a team of advanced graduates at a prominent university. They met all IRB requirements for human subjects approval but failed to negotiate their purposes with school personnel and never built a transpar-ent and ongoing relationship; thus, teachers and school leaders often were offended by both actions and conclusions of the researchers. They felt that the researchers had summarily misrepresented them and that they had no input into the interpretation. The result was a request from one participating school to withdraw from the study, a right they remembered was promised in the informed consent agreement. (This example is more fully described and analyzed in Rallis, 2010.)

Respecting people—whoever they are, wherever they are—takes place in every aspect of research and is seen in the everyday encounters of researchers with, in these examples, adolescents, campesinos, teachers, or principals. Respecting people can be quite challenging when you don't understand that asking them a question that is strange and that puts them off

Relational matters matter. ← (4)

may well be *dis*respectful. To end this example, we note that the consultants may well have sacrificed the validity of the data by insisting on questions that were essentially meaningless to the campesinos.

Given these observations, we argue that the trustworthiness, or rigor, of a study should depend not just on whether the researcher got the technical matters right—whether about instrumentation or the protection of human subjects. Trustworthiness should also be judged by how well the researcher got the relational matters right. We hold that relational matters are present in all research, whether archival research, secondary analyses of large-scale databases, survey research, long-term ethnography, or quasi-experimental and experimental research. The intensity and duration of the relations vary, as does the ethical obligation of the researcher.

Research studies can and should be designed and conducted in ways that benefit participants. These benefits can take various forms. Some studies, such as policy or program evaluations, express the benefits as program improvement. Many identify the intended recipients of the benefits: for example, "Principals can use the resulting information to facilitate teacher teams." In much research, benefits to participants are implicit and often unintended: For example, an interviewee learns something positive and important about herself during the conversation, or participants feel honored that their stories are told. In all cases, benefits begin with the relationships built around the research.

critique question self-reflect. Your particip and question.

We argue that these relational matters are central not only to ethical considerations but also to judgments about the overall trustworthiness of a study. Thus, we define trustworthiness as composed of both *competent practice* and *ethical considerations for the participants*, with an underlying demand that the relational matters involved in *any* research be foregrounded and privileged (Rossman & Rallis, 2012). As Davies and Dodd (2002) note:

> Ethics are an essential part of rigorous research. Ethics are more than a
> set of principles or abstract rules that sit as an overarching entity guiding

our research. . . . Ethics exist in our actions and in our ways of doing and practicing our research; we perceive ethics to be always in progress, never to be taken for granted, flexible, and responsive to change. (p. 281)

Ethical practice, then, is a conscious and continuous process that we suggest begins with relationships. We won't pretend that building ethical relationships with participants is easy or instantaneous, but we do believe that it becomes easier when we articulate (at least explicitly to ourselves) the moral principles we intend to use. For example, we recall the study where a university research team (consisting of a PI and five graduate students) never dialogued with the people in the selected study schools in order to establish common purposes; they made explicit neither their principles nor the potential benefits to the participants. Had they done so, the schools might not have closed their doors to the team, as they eventually did, or new agreements might have been negotiated. At the end, because no shared principles existed, the schools felt the weight of the research burden—they discovered that the researchers' goals differed from their own, so the benefit they experienced was limited.

Our point is that a researcher's moral principles, explicit or not, drive research practice and affect the study's trustworthiness. Recognizing the driving principles is both critical and complicated because not all moral principles are compatible, and contradictions even lie within some. Moreover, the researcher is challenged to translate abstract principles into practical actions. Certain ethical theories provide the bridge between moral principles and practical actions; to these we now turn.

ETHICAL THEORIES

Consequentialist ethical theories rest on a set of moral principles that focus on outcomes, on results of actions. Any particular action is neither intrinsically good nor bad; rather, it is good or bad because of its results in a particular context—its consequences. If the end has value, the means are less important. The best known example of a consequentialist ethical theory is *utilitarianism,* which would suggest that a researcher design a study that likely results in the greatest good for the greatest number. A researcher who is guided by an *ethic of consequences* (the basic idea underlying utilitarianism) would seek to maximize the benefits of the study to participants, policy, perhaps even society.

Nonconsequentialist ethical theories, on the other hand, recognize universal standards to guide all behavior, regardless of the consequences in a specific context. Thus, if a decision or action is wrong, it must be wrong in all possible contexts. Two nonconsequentialist theories are the *ethic of individual rights and responsibilities* and *the ethic of justice*. The first upholds the unconditional worth of and equal respect to which all human beings are entitled. This ethic judges actions by the degree to which they respect a person's rights, not by its outcomes or consequences. Each person must be treated as an end in herself, not as a means to an end. The protection of these rights may not be denied, even for the greatest good for the greatest number. *Ethics of justice* go beyond individual rights and responsibilities to espouse the redistribution of resources and opportunities to achieve equity above equality. Principles of fairness and equity are used to judge which actions are right and wrong. The goal is to ensure that everyone is better off, even though the allocation of some benefit may differ. Such apparently unequal treatment is justified because not attending to the least is to hurt the whole.

Principles of justice and individual rights consider questions of power and representation: Who defines what is right in a given situation? Whose values are used in defining what is right? Are all voices given opportunity to be heard? Are benefits likely to accrue to the most vulnerable as a result of participating? According to Rawls (1971), the benefit or welfare of the least advantaged, not that of the majority or average, must drive any action. His view maintains that improving the welfare of the least advantaged ultimately benefits everyone because the communal resources of society and future generations will grow.

While these two major sets of theories offer guidance for the researcher–participant relationship, other perspectives more explicitly situate morality within the context and relationship. For example, *communitarianism* (MacIntyre, 1981) acknowledges that communities differ on what is morally good or right. Researchers may find that not all people within their research setting share fundamental values and that those values may conflict with the researchers' own values. Within this perspective, the thorny issue arises of whose values define the research, guide decisions, and shape interpretations. In other words, whose values are dominant, which voices determine what is ethical, and what happens to those voices that are silenced? Our character Reilly would argue that a postmodern response posits that power and dominant versions of "truth" shape the relationships (Foucault, 1977).

Still, none of these theories or perspectives may be practically helpful to get researchers through ethical challenges because, as theories, they are necessarily abstract. As Noddings notes, "Ethical decisions must be made in caring interactions with those affected by the discussion. Indeed, it is exactly in the most difficult situations that principles fail us" (1995, p. 187). She articulates an alternative and potentially quite powerful way to conceptualize the moral and ethical aspects of research that spotlights the relationship itself. The *ethics of care* emphasizes concrete circumstances over abstract principles: What does *this* person need in *this* moment? "Our goodness and our growth are inextricably bound to that of others we encounter. As researchers, we are as dependent on our [participants] as they are on us" (Noddings, 1995, p. 196). The aim is to build the mutual respect necessary for a reciprocal relationship: "One must meet the other in caring. From this requirement there is no escape for one who would be moral" (Noddings, 1984, p. 201). Mutual care and respect can bridge the gap between the purposes and needs of both members in the relationship. Thus, the ethic of caring honors the moral interdependence of people—relational matters— rather than focusing on the individual as a moral agent or on mere procedures that attempt to police those relationships. We suggest that care theory, with its emphasis on relationships, can connect people and principles, providing a practical framework for making moral decisions that a qualitative researcher will encounter. Ethical research demands *caring reflexivity* (Rallis & Rossman, 2010).

Consider possible studies our characters could propose to explore their interests:

• *Kevin* seeks to learn interventions that can address learning problems that adolescent boys experience. His expressed aim is to find programs that help the most boys; thus, he has articulated a consequentialist ethic, utilitarianism. Raul points out that a program designed with the multitude in mind may overlook or damage a small subset of boys, thus violating their rights as individuals, suggesting a more nonconsequentialist ethic. Samira questions whether Kevin ought to look at what the boys need in particular contexts, with a focus on how the boys relate to the learning activity; her ideas reflect an ethic of care.

• *Martina* proposes to look at inequities in opportunity for the village orphans, revealing either an ethic of individual rights or an ethic of justice. Reilly elaborates on an ethic of justice with a critical turn as he encourages

Martina to emphasize the power imbalances that arise from the interventions brought by nongovernmental organizations and the need to address these inequities. Kevin reminds her that all the children in the village could become orphans from HIV/AIDS, and so wonders why not seek interventions that address the greatest number of children, whatever their current status (utilitarianism again).

ETHICS AND REFLEXIVITY

Clearly, there are no prescribed procedures or techniques for engaging with "ethically important moments" (Guillemin & Gillam, 2004). However, we have argued that methodological deliberations demand consideration of the ethical. As well, these deliberations honor relationships over procedures. Perhaps most important in making ethical judgments is the need to recognize that such judgments are not merely matters of personal opinion and preference; they are, rather, judgments that affect more than the researcher and, therefore, must be transparent. We argue that the better our ethical reasoning, the better our decisions and, ultimately, the more trustworthy our research.

As Guillemin and Gillam (2004) point out, reflexivity is essential for trustworthiness in research. Reflexivity is "looking at yourself making sense of how someone else makes sense of her world" (Rossman & Rallis, 2012, p. 47). Reflexivity demands the ongoing interrogation of: What do I see? How and why do I see this? How might others see it? What does it mean to me? To others? Reflexivity *is* relational—it recognizes that the researcher and the participants are involved in continual and changing interaction. The researcher asks: What might be possible consequences of my relationship with participants? Of my interpretations? What rights of participants might I violate or what potential harms might result? Are the participants likely to benefit in any way, and are they likely to agree on the benefit? To be trustworthy, the relationship must be ethical, that is, consciously guided by explicit moral principles. Ultimately, to produce knowledge that can be used for improvement, the reflexive process invites a researcher to identify her ethical perspective: What are my values? What rules or standards apply? What moral principles guide my decisions? Equally critical is that the researcher question her actions: Do I act according to my principles?

> Be reflexive about ethics . . . and people.

Conscious reflexivity driven by one's ethical stance offers the antidote to harm. This reflection on and into action serves "partly to check that the researcher's practice is actually embodying his or her principles; in addition, this allows the researcher to become aware of situations where following the theoretical position may not be the best course and may not best uphold the interests of his or her participants" (Guillemin & Gillam, 2004, p. 276). Reflexivity then recognizes the import of both principles and the unique context of the relationship, connecting principles and context, providing a practical framework for making moral decisions. As we argued earlier, ethical research demands *caring reflexivity.*

A complex example illustrates the points of this chapter (the following vignette captures the experience of Habibullah Wajdi, a doctoral student at the University of Massachusetts):

> **Setting the scene:** Wajdi, a doctoral student in international education, is from Afghanistan and is passionate about improving both access to and quality of schools in his country. He argues that deep and lasting change can occur only locally—that *hashar,* a call for collective action, is a centuries-old traditional norm that is still a common practice for making changes in rural communities today. Wajdi sees abundant examples of hashar for construction of mosques, crop harvesting, cleaning the irrigation canals, shoveling roofs and pathways, digging *karezes* (irrigation wells), contribution of land, and sharing of land for collective good. He argues that this collective action contributes to social capital, and he wonders if this same force could work to improve schools. The purpose of his dissertation study, then, is to understand the forms of social capital that exist in rural communities and to explore the linkages between rural schools and prevailing social capital in rural areas of Afghanistan.
>
> One source of data Wajdi uses is interviews with village elders. What follows is an excerpt from his dialogue with an older woman, Bibi Amana (for her respect and her pilgrimage she is called Bibi Hajani), in the village, during which he seeks to establish informed consent. He is aware that obtaining a signature is unlikely, but he feels comfortable talking with the elder about his purposes and her role. We enter the conversation just after Wajdi has explained his purpose and that he is doing the study for his degree from an American university. The conversation is in Pashtu and has been translated.

W: Bibi Hajani! You be never tired! Be well and safe! [a traditional common greeting, which has positive tone for starting a long conversation; maybe similar to "How are you?" or "How have you been," etc.]

A: Welcome! May you come again and again! Live long my child. [a traditional way of replying to greetings; sets the reciprocity and positive feelings]

W: May you be blessed that you are willing to give me some of your time. I am hoping that you will speak with me about the village. Many thanks!

A: *(pouring cups of green tea)* Thank you for coming to my home. I am happy that you want to know about this humble village. But why do you want to talk with me? I am just an old woman.

W: With your age, you have experience and wisdom. You are Bibi Hajani—you have seen the world. The people recognize you as an honored leader of this village. Your knowledge of the people and what happens in the village is great. I can learn much from you.

A: Perhaps I do have knowledge you may want. But why should I talk with you? What will you do with my words?

W: As I told you, I am a student at a university in the United States. I will write a long paper—my dissertation—about what I learn in your village, and in the other villages I visit.

A: Who will read this paper?

W: My professors and other students. If the paper is good enough, I hope to publish it so that many people will read it and maybe some will use what I learn to help us improve our schools.

A: That is fine, but what we need first is help in cleaning the irrigation canals so we can harvest better crops. Schools can come later. Can your people help us with water?

W: I cannot promise that help with water. I cannot even promise that anyone will help with schools. I can only try to write what I hear you say and then hope that others will read it and act in ways that will help.

A: Der Sha—well enough. You tell me you want to learn about schools in the village. That is the business of the Malem [teacher] and Mullah [religious leader]. You can talk with them. *(Smiles.)*

W: Yes, I will, but I want also to hear what you have to say. You can tell me who goes to school and what you think of the schools. I will honor and respect your words.

A: Yes, but what if I will say things the Malem and Mullah will not. But maybe you will just tell them what I say. They will be offended. That might not be good for harmony in the village.

W: I give you my word that I will not go to them with what you say. I do not need to tell them your words. Still, you know that I will write your words in my paper for the university. How do you feel about your words being written and shared with people outside the village?

A: I might like that. I might not. It depends on how you write my words. How can I know what you do with my words?

W: Would you allow me to tape record what you say? (*Describes the process and shows her the recorder*)

A: No, I will not allow that. But you can bring to me the writing you make of my words. I cannot read, but perhaps one of the schoolchildren can read them to me.

Wajdi and Bibi Amana continue to talk about how she can know what he writes and what purpose his study will serve. Wajdi is careful not to make promises he cannot keep. She agrees to talk with him the next day.

We hope you can see how a researcher's daily practice is filled with moments that demand decisions—ethical choices grounded in moral reasoning. Implicit in systematic inquiry is transparent decision making, and each decision will in some way touch and affect the study participants, whether their participation is face to face, through a survey, or indirectly through a dataset. Thus, while procedures set a standard, relationships determine trustworthiness. What makes any given decision ethical is not that the researcher follows any particular procedure, but that her choices are a product of her reflexive moral reasoning. Because people—human beings—are central to social science research, the participants and the researcher are morally interdependent. Recognizing this connection, the ethical and competent researcher cares about her participants; she builds and explores relationships—in whatever form they may take—that honor and protect the realities of her participants' lives. Working with and through these relationships, she informs the research questions; she discovers and learns. The ethical and competent researcher practices reflexivity every day.

Learning Activity 4.1. "The Moral Fix": A Debate

This activity draws on the classic reading "The Moral Fix" by John Van Maanen (1983). In his research with police squadrons, Van Maanen "assumed" the persona of a rookie cop. He went on patrol with them, ate with them, and witnessed what might be seen as brutality with them. In this article, he discusses his choice *not* to intervene in events of brutality and the reasoning behind that choice.

Divide your group in half. If you have more than 10 members, break into smaller groups such as your triads. Assign a position to each half of the group: one agrees with Van Maanen's decisions, the other disagrees. Each group prepares an argument grounded in moral principles and ethical research practice. Remember that ethical choices involve weighing often conflicting sets of obligations to various individuals or groups: to participants, to society, to knowledge, to a funding agency, to oneself as a researcher and human being.

Take 15 minutes to develop the key points in your argument. In classic debate style, the group who agrees with Van Maanen's choice presents its case. Then the group that disagrees presents its argument. Each presentation should be no more than 10 minutes. Rebuttals are then given by the proponent group, followed by rebuttals by the opposition.

The strength of this activity lies in each group arguing cogently and passionately for the position you are assigned. At first glance, many disagree with Van Maanen's choices, but if you consider carefully the circumstances of the police and the expectations in which he had participated (and helped create), your assessment of his decision may be more subtle.

Learning Activity 4.2. What Would You Do?

The following are examples of troubling circumstances that arose during the conduct of two actual research projects. In small groups (your triad is ideal for this activity), identify the issues and the relevant ethical principles. Given these issues, would you consider that the studies will be rigorous and will result in credible findings? Provide a rationale for your choice. What would you do if you were in either of these situations?

An Evaluation of a Citizen Change Initiative

A team of evaluators was contracted to assess an ambitious citizen-driven change initiative in five Latin American countries. The initiative, Podemos Hacerlo, had the goal of fostering agency—self-efficacy—among ordinary citizens such that they would feel empowered to advocate with government officials about their access to and the quality of basic services. The initiative was quite bold in scope and drew on partnerships with various organizations and networks for implementation.

The evaluation design called, in part, for conducting a nationally representative, randomly sampled household survey in the five countries. The evaluation team called on expert consultants to help design the household survey. Issues arose at a workshop with the team and the consultants where specific questionnaire items were discussed. One member of the evaluation team came from a village in a very rural area in the country where the workshop was held and spoke the local language where field testing was planned. His cultural sensitivities and linguistic knowledge were crucial for developing questions that would be meaningful and appropriate for campesinos. However, he felt that many of the consultants' questions would be meaningless to campesinos because their theoretical framework was Western, individualistic, and grounded in an orientation to change and a future that was not congruent with values and beliefs in that context. He argued quite eloquently that these be changed prior to field testing. However, his expertise, local knowledge, and critical wisdom were ignored by the consultants.

Despite the evaluation team's best efforts, preliminary field testing of the questionnaire (a common and crucially important practice in questionnaire development) was scheduled to take place in a rural town and its surrounding villages not far from the capital city. The evaluation team observed that the campesinos found questions such as "When do you feel most like yourself?" and "What would you like to change in your life?" baffling and, in some cases, insulting. Many of the questions made the campesinos feel inadequate and frustrated (because the questions were meaningless).

A Study of Adolescents at Risk

A student in psychology was an RA on a study to measure the effects of a particular intervention with adolescents who abused alcohol. Because the study was conducted in a research university, IRB approval was required. As the RA, the student was charged with completing the varied and numerous forms that included guarantees of confidentiality and protection from harm. The required procedures were extensive and thorough; the RA fully complied, and the study received approval.

Very quickly, the study ran into problems with recruitment. The participants were minors, so parental consent was required, but many potential participants did not want to reveal their alcohol use to parents. Because the number of participants was not high enough to meet the design projections, the PI demanded more effort to bring in participants and even recommended that the criteria for selection (e.g., participants had to be under a certain weight, could not be hard-drug users, could not report being depressed) be relaxed. The RA wondered how he could increase participation while still ensuring that participants were not exposed to possible harm.

The RA also was disturbed when he heard secretaries talking about a participant and again when he witnessed a list of those who had not been selected being passed to another study. He considered these actions to be violations of the promised confidentiality. As the weeks passed, the RA began to realize that much of his efforts to comply with the IRB procedures had little connection to reality. Moreover, he realized that what he considered to be ethical violations also compromised the study: How could they claim findings were valid and reliable if participants did not even meet the study criteria?

FOR FURTHER READING

American Educational Research Association. (2011). *AERA code of ethics.* Retrieved October 1, 2011, from *www.aera.net/EthicsCode.htm.*

American Evaluation Association. (2004). *Guiding principles for evaluators.* Retrieved October 1, 2011, from *www.eval.org/publications/guidingprinciples. asp.*

American Sociological Association. (1991). *ASA code of ethics.* Retrieved October 1, 2011, from *www.asanet.org/about/ethics.cfm.*

Berry, D. M. (2004). Internet research: Privacy, ethics and alienation: An open source approach. *Internet Research, 14*(4), 323–332.

Chadwick, R., ten Have, H., & Meslin, E. M. (2011). *The Sage handbook of health care ethics.* Thousand Oaks, CA: Sage.

Howe, K. R., & Moses, M. S. (1999). Ethics in educational research. *Review of Research in Education, 24*, 21–59.

↪ Hutchins, P. (2002). *Ethics of inquiry: Issues in the scholarship of teaching and learning*. Menlo Park, CA: Carnegie Foundation for the Advancement of Teaching.

↪ Israel, M., & Hay, I. (2006). *Research ethics for social scientists*. London: Sage.

↪ Macrina, F. L. (2005). *Scientific integrity: Text and cases in responsible conduct of research* (3rd ed.). Washington, DC: ASM Press.

↪ Mauthner, M. L., Mauthner, M., Birch, M., & Jessop, J. (2002). *Ethics in qualitative research*. Thousand Oaks, CA: Sage.

↪ Mertens, D. H., & Ginsberg, P. E. (Eds.). (2009). *The handbook of social research ethics*. Thousand Oaks, CA: Sage.

↪ Morris, M. (Ed.). (2007). *Evaluation ethics for best practice: Cases and commentaries*. New York: Guilford Press.

↪ Sikes, P., Nixon, J., & Carr, W. (Eds.). (2003). *The moral foundations of educational research: Knowledge, inquiry and values*. Maidenhead, UK: Open University Press.

CHAPTER 5

Constructing Conceptual Frameworks
Building the Route

✸ *Critical Questions to Guide Your Reading*

➥ *What is a conceptual framework? (remembering)*

➥ *What is the relationship between a literature review and a conceptual framework? (analyzing)*

➥ *What role does theory play in a conceptual framework? (analyzing)*

➥ *How does a central argument develop from a conceptual framework? (analyzing)*

➥ *Who are the members of my community of practice? (applying)*

➥ *Who is my main audience? (applying)*

➥ *What "currents of thought" are most relevant for my inquiry project? (evaluating)*

➥ *How might I effectively organize my discussion of the literature? (applying)*

Dialogue 5. Grappling with a Conceptual Framework

Professor Bettara asked the students to get into groups of three—their triads. The purpose of the exercise was to share with one another their initial thinking about the argument they want to make—their intuitive locating—and "currents of thought" that might support their argument. Each member was told to speak for no more than 5 minutes, with no questions from their partners. After speaking, the other members could ask questions. Bettara stressed that the partners could only ask questions; no reactions or comments were to be allowed. Martina, Samira, and Reilly pulled their chairs together to form a triad.

SAMIRA: I really wouldn't know where to begin. I only know I'm interested in social justice. Why don't you start, Martina? You seem to at least have a focus.

MARTINA: Yes, but this is very difficult for me! I've been doing this work for the Rainbow Fellowship that is gathering information about what's happening with AIDS-affected children in my village. I'm not a physician, so I don't know much about the disease; all I know is that many, many children are heading up households and caring for younger kids. And what makes it such a tragedy is that the kids who take on this responsibility for their siblings cannot make it to school. They get trapped. Sometimes other family members help out, but everyone is facing really difficult times. I'm just not sure what relevant research and theories might help me build a conceptual framework.

REILLY: Oh, but there's the whole critique of development that you should use. It's loaded with insights about why there is still such great poverty in your kind of country.

SAMIRA: (*Interrupting*) Hang on there. First, Bettara said we could only ask questions. And second, what do you mean when you say "your kind of country?" Sounds pretty arrogant to me.

REILLY: Hey, wait a sec. I'm just trying to help her out.

SAMIRA: Then let's hear what Martina's thinking.

MARTINA: OK, I'll go on. I've got a lot of statistics about poverty levels and the incidence of HIV/AIDS. And I believe there is something about the intersection of economic opportunity, politics, and AIDS, but I'm not sure. I need to look into this more deeply.

REILLY: What is going on politically?

MARTINA: Good question. The former president was from a different tribe than my village. Over the years, they never received any "benefits" from his presidency; in fact, they suffered while other areas of the country were given preference. I'm just not sure how to tie this into my interest in the children who are heads of household or to turn it into an argument.

SAMIRA: Wow. That sounds like something I'd be interested in. I'd want to argue that national policies are inequitable and unjust. Can you talk some more about how the president's decisions affected your village?

Martina went on to describe, in some detail, how previously enacted policies shaped her community's access to health care, economic opportunities through building good roads, and pastoral care through religious organizations. Although she had only begun to articulate an argument and conceptual framework—and was not even sure that it was the "correct" one—she had the beginnings of a roadmap that could guide further explorations in the literature.

Note that in this activity Bettara insisted that students only ask questions of one another; they were not supposed to offer comments. We invite you to think about why this might be a useful pedagogical strategy. Also note that our "bad boy" Reilly was unable to abide by this directive. What is important, however, is that he was "disciplined" by members of his community of practice rather than by the professor. This is important because it represents the assumption, on the part of two members of the triad, of responsibility for their own learning and that of their colleagues.

As this dialogue depicts, beginning to build a conceptual framework and an argument that will guide an inquiry project is challenging intellectual work. In fact, we claim that it is the *most* challenging—and most important—aspect of designing a project. It entails iterative processes, that is, recursive activities that both build on each other and loop back to revisit assumptions (remember double-loop learning in Chapter 3). Conceptual frameworks can fruitfully be thought of as composing the *what* of the study (Marshall & Rossman, 2011; Rossman & Rallis, 2012), where the "substantive focus of the study" is described (Marshall & Rossman, 2011, p. 6); these ideas were introduced briefly in Chapter 2. The design for conducting the inquiry (discussed in Chapter 6) is *how* you plan to implement the inquiry and follows from the *what*. Both are interrelated sets of considerations; here, we separate out the conceptual framing but remember that considering *how* you might implement the inquiry will recursively shape the *what*.

Major activities in developing a conceptual framework include identifying and interrogating your personal perspectives; considering a variety of strands of theorizing and research; determining whether these would be generative for the project; exploring them in depth. What does this mean for you? First, this entails asking yourself where you stand on the issue, what your intuitive perspective is: "You need to determine *how* you see and how *you* see" (Schram, 2006, p. 39). Think about the sets of assumptions about ontology and epistemology discussed in Chapter 2; draw on these to create a more developed "research perspective" or "research orientation," as we have mentioned. Second, conceptualizing entails reading openly and widely; more reading; talking to your community of practice; and then more focused reading, this time with a critical eye. The virtue of this early exploration is that it helps you come in touch with the strands of thinking—the "currents of thought" (Schram, 2006, p. 63)—that will be meaningful for framing the project.

A note here: A conceptual framework cannot be fully developed until you have immersed yourself in relevant theorizing and research; however, you will be lost in reading the literature unless you enter with an intuitive sense of what might be the key elements of the conceptual framework, what might be called "sensitizing concepts" (Blumer, 1954, p. 7), to give you direction. This chapter focuses on this intuitive locating, on reading relevant literature, and ways these are brought together to become the guiding framework for the project.

At this point, you may be asking yourself several questions: What is a "conceptual framework?" What does "conceptualizing" mean? Why is it central to inquiry? Why an argument? How does building an argument fit with the conceptual framework? What role does a literature review play? This chapter explores these questions.

WHAT IS A CONCEPTUAL FRAMEWORK?

A conceptual framework is a structure that organizes the currents of thought that provide focus and direction to an inquiry. It is the organization of ideas—the central concepts from theory, key findings from research, policy statements, professional wisdom—that will guide the project. Framework

= organization or structure. Conceptual = concerning thoughts, ideas, perceptions, or theories. The framework emerges from wide and intensive reading of relevant literature and links your project to ongoing conversations in your field, thereby establishing parameters: what your focus is, and what it is *not*. It also provides direction for the research questions you pose, for design decisions, and for preliminary analytic strategies. As such, a well-developed and integrated conceptual framework distinguishes a thoughtful inquiry project from those that are impoverished, at least intellectually. Most important, a conceptual framework provides coherence to your thoughts, making it easier to convey "how and why your ideas matter relative to some larger body of ideas embodied in the research, writings, and experiences of others" (Schram, 2006, p. 58). As noted earlier, this is often the most challenging aspect of inquiry; unfortunately, it is often misunderstood, glided over, or given short shrift. In their article "Overlooking the Conceptual Framework," Leshem and Trafford (2007) describe how research candidates are not well taught about how to develop interesting conceptual frameworks and how little attention these are given in research methods texts.

As you come to know your perspective, identify your interests, and read what others have written on the topic, you are conceptualizing. The ultimate goal here is to "produce a coherent, focused, integrative, and contestable argument that is comprehensible to readers who are not directly acquainted with your topic" (Schram, 2006, p. 63). The framework acts as a kind of boundary for the inquiry. We think of conceptual frameworks as comprising three interlinked elements: your perspective, relevant research, and generative theories or theoretical constructs.

Building a conceptual framework starts with you, your knowledge and interests that may emerge from past experiences and study. You ask: What do I care about sufficiently to learn about in more depth? What do I know about this from my own experience? Why is this topic important to me? How do I feel about the issue or topic? How can this interest—my passion—become a feasible topic for an inquiry project? The answers to these questions contribute to the sensitizing concepts that "draw attention to important features of social interaction and provide guidelines for research in specific settings" (Bowen, 2006, p. 3). These concepts "offer ways of seeing, organizing, and understanding experience" (Charmaz, 2003, p. 259) and "suggest directions along which to look" (Blumer, 1954, p. 7) for currents of thought you will need to explore. Because we are thinking beings—*Homo sapiens sapiens*—we carry these interests, preferences, and interpretations of experience in our heads, and inquiry begins with such concepts, whether we have made them explicit or are even aware of them. However, systematic research requires you to be aware of and state them. As you begin to focus what may be a diffuse set of interests into an inquiry topic, you are beginning to develop an intuitive framing. As you explore and answer these questions for yourself, you articulate central assertions or claims that are grounded in your interests. You thus make the conceptual framework *yours*—an understandable and integrated context for your inquiry project.

2   A second element is the literature—what is already known and talked about concerning the topic. You will discover and critically read the research, policy writings, reports about practice, evaluations, essays, perhaps newspaper articles, maybe even popular communication on the topic. You ask: What questions have been explored that relate to mine? What research can I build on? What have "experts" said about this topic? What is the discourse in the public domain? No matter what your general area of interest, some research is likely to have been conducted. We are quite suspicious when students claim that there has been no research that is related to their inquiry projects. This is just not the case! Although there may be no research that has been done on this specific topic, with this particular population or sample, using the research methods you envision, there is *related research* that you must be draw on to demonstrate your familiarity with the currents of thought in your chosen field.

3   A third element is the theory or theoretical constructs that you have determined will be generative in grounding the project. Many of the research reports that you read will have theoretical groundings, so pay attention to these as you read the research. Here you ask: What theoretical ideas or concepts usefully provide direction for my inquiry project? A word here about theory, an often misused and misunderstood term: A theory is a set of propositions that underlie, explain, and predict phenomena; it is a model of some aspect of reality. However, a theory does not have to be universally accepted; a theory can be viewed as a set of working understandings or hypotheses (Weiss, 1998). Many references to theory imply what we call small-"*t*" theory—hunches or an intuitive set of ideas believed to guide actions. We all carry *theories* around in our heads, theories we use on a daily basis. For example, a small "*t*" about instruction in the college classroom might lead us to modify a teaching strategy based on the prediction that this change could lead to better student performance. We are thus "theorizing" about teaching, based on professional wisdom and experience. If we are good scientists, we gather data about this new strategy, remaining

open to failure, partial success, or outstanding success. In the case of the first two, we might then revise our teaching "theory."

Theory with a capital *T* refers to an accepted "set of assumptions, axioms, propositions, or definitions that form a coherent and unified description of a circumstance, situation, or phenomenon" (Burke, 2009, p. 62). These Theories are labeled (e.g., self-efficacy) and often attributed to an individual or group of individuals (e.g., Erickson's [1959] Identity Theory or Levinson's [1978, 1996] Adult Development Theory). Both Theory and theories contribute to a generative conceptual framework, one that can be considered *foundational* (i.e., based in theory). Both kinds of theory serve to connect focused ideas—for example, HIV/AIDS-affected children in Kenya—to larger ones—postcolonial theories—and provide a direction for analysis. Note that we write "provide a *direction* for analysis." This is important because good inquiry demands openness to the unexpected: "Theory can provide perspective and suggest pattern, but it need not define what you can see" (Schram, 2006, p. 60).

Figure 5.1 depicts these key elements. Note that these contribute to the conceptual framework and also provide preliminary guidance for an analytic

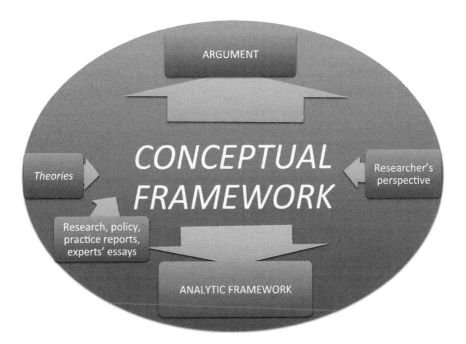

FIGURE 5.1. Conceptual and analytic frameworks.

framework—key concepts and hypotheses that will guide data analysis as you move through your inquiry cycle.

Thus, the conceptual framework provides the basis for a coherent study. It connects the *what* with the *how* of the inquiry. In short, you conceptualize the *what* by embedding your ideas and questions in a larger pool of ideas and questions: What experiences have you had with the question or problem? What are related concepts? What have others already learned about the issues? What research has already been conducted? What Theories might inform the ideas? You are making an argument and positioning it on the terrain of your journey. The framework also links to the design for the study, ensuring that the approach and methods are coherent and flow logically from the framework, and provides a preliminary map for analyzing the data, that is, a preliminary analytic (as depicted in Figure 5.1).

We now present an extended example developed from the conceptual framework of a former student, Aysen Kose (2010). Her conceptual framework encompasses the elements (argument; researcher's perspective; Theoretical frames; research, policy, and practice reports; analytic framework) in Figure 5.1. Lest you feel overwhelmed by the following example, we assure you that the work represents more than a semester in the *Introduction to Inquiry* course; in fact, we draw on Kose's dissertation to describe and illustrate the process:

AYSEN'S CONCEPTUALIZING PROCESS

School Counselors' Leadership Practices
through the Lens of Distributed Leadership

Personal perspective (experiences and values): Aysen, a former school counselor in Turkey, was frustrated with the limitations on her role that required her to work with individual students who experienced problems. She saw this approach as situating the problem in the student, not in the context of the school where the student experienced the problem. She believed that usually it isn't the student who needs fixing, it is the system, so she asked: Why don't counselors take on more systemic roles within the school? What factors support or inhibit counselors working with the system as well as with individual students?

Research and policy: Through her reading and classes, Aysen learned about a new vision for school counselors that drew on concepts of advocacy, leadership, teamwork and collaboration, accountability, use of data, and systemic change. The new vision for school counselors requires that counselors take leadership roles to become advocates and change agents for the success of all students and must align comprehensive counseling programs toward the mission of the schools. Her review of the literature contrasted the old image of the counselor's role (works to help individual students; operates in a "counseling silo" within the school) with the new (works to change the system rather than the individual student; is integral to the operation of the school as a whole).

Theoretical constructs: Aysen's reading led her to explore Theories of leadership and change. Specifically, she discovered several useful and relevant theories: organizational structure (e.g., Argyris & Schön, 1978; Elmore, 2000), distributed leadership (e.g., Spillane, 2004), and change agency and systemic change (e.g. Carr-Chellman, 1998; Senge, 1994). These contributed to her articulation of an argument to guide her study (and eventually served to guide her analysis).

Argument: The new vision requires school counselors to serve all students, not just those who need individual assistance; thus, school counselors are expected to provide leadership not only at an individual level but also at the school system level. The new school counselor will be a change agent, a proactive participant in school improvement efforts. For the counselor to operate systemically and collaboratively, school leadership activities must be distributed across all members of the organization.

Research question: How do school counselors enact overall school leadership practice for schoolwide improvement?

1. What formal and informal organizational routines allow school counselors to take on leadership roles? How do school counselors contribute to constructive leadership practices through those routines?

2. What activities do school counselors implement that demonstrate the new vision of school counseling? How have these activities changed over the last 8 years?

Analytic framework: Aysen's data analysis followed several phases. According to *distributed leadership theory*, leadership practice is shaped through social interactions and routines, which are observable practices. Thus, she began by identifying *formal* and *informal* routines and events in which the school counselors participated and by organizing them in a table according to purpose, persons involved (leaders and followers), role distribution, tools used, and who called the meeting. Next, she coded the events and routines for characteristics using categories from her conceptual framework, such as systemic, focused around single student, demand driven, structural, counselor initiated. Her next phase coded the counselors' actions within the routines: specific tasks, roles, times and places, substance. Finally, she sought to identify core patterns (or lack of) across the routines.

Through your conceptual framework, you explicate and ground the perspective *you* have developed toward the issue: Who are you in relation to this question, this problem? Why do you want to inform it, to address it? How does your focus link to larger issues? Who else is interested? We have found it useful to use the metaphor of a "lens" for this. The metaphor captures both *what* you see and *how* you will see it. Cameras differ and capture different aspects of the social world based on, for example, the photographer's perspective—his or her position—as well as camera settings—shutter speed, lighting, wide angle or zoom, color or black and white. All these elements shape the resulting picture, just as with inquiry. Think of the conceptual framework as the sum of these elements: the perspective that you bring—your camera, if you will—to better understanding, and perhaps hoping to change, some aspect of the social world that intrigues you. Overall, the conceptual framework captures the complex deductive–inductive reasoning that goes into framing the study; it brings together the abstract and the concrete, the general and the specific.

> Conceptual framework
> = your lens.

In summary, conceptual frameworks serve many purposes; they:

- *Construct* the argument;
- *Describe* and *map* the topic of interest;

- *Identify* key epistemological assumptions and personal or professional interests—your intellectual orientation;
- *Situate* the study in the ongoing scholarly conversations about the topic—the various research discourses;
- *Recognize* potential contributions of the study to knowledge (the literature, theory, policy discussions, and/or issues of practice);
- *Develop* "sensitizing concepts" (Blumer, 1954, p. 7);
- *Suggest* (sometimes preliminary) analytic variables, categories, and/or themes;
- *Sharpen* the focus;
- *Generate* hypotheses and/or research questions; and
- *Provide* direction for analysis.

As noted previously, developing a conceptual framework entails critically examining all three elements (your perspective, Theory, and related research) for their relevance, insightfulness, credibility, and usefulness. Although personal or professional experience (discussed in greater detail later) can provide the wellspring for interest in a topic, you must subject that experience to serious examination and critique. Your experience does *not* generalize to the world.

BUILDING AN ARGUMENT

Thinking about conceptualizing as creating an argument helps to situate *you* in the topic. In essence, you put forward a point of view and a context for the inquiry in which the problem or interest or issue and the reasons and strategies for pursuing it are convincing. You are making a case and building a logic to support that case. We suggest that many communications (an e-mail, an advertisement, even a love letter) can be viewed as arguments in the sense that they want to convince the reader of something: that the work needs to be completed, that the product is worth buying, that your feelings are valuable. So too a conceptual framework is making a central argument: This topic or focus is well framed by drawing on X, Y, and Z traditions in scholarly writing. The conceptual framework clarifies this perspective at the

> **Arguments are meant to convince the reader.**

outset, stating it clearly so that readers can understand your map and agree, disagree, or suggest modifications. For example, Martina's emerging argument might be stated as: *As a consequence of the HIV/AIDS pandemic, many children have been orphaned, and many have become heads of their households. They cannot attend school; they are burdened with caring for younger siblings or relatives; they are unable to find sufficient food and clean water for themselves and those in their care. All too often governments turn a deaf ear to their plight and have not enacted policies that treat these children equitably and beneficially, ensuring a social network that supports the children's well-being.* The problem is clear: Too many households are headed by children. Martina's passion is clear: This is a deeply disturbing circumstance. And the framing literature is suggested: government policies and programs.

To build an argument is to state how you understand a phenomenon—your central claim or thesis—that is supported with reasons and evidence; considerations of alternative views; and putting forward a rationale. Developing a convincing and credible argument is central to your work as a scholar, as an inquirer. Why do we emphasize "convincing"? Much writing at the graduate level—scholarly term papers, proposals for research, theses and dissertations—depends on an argument and supporting evidence that *convinces* readers of the plausibility of your argument. Imagine a thesis or dissertation proposal defense. And note that these are typically referred to as "defenses," whether in the natural or social sciences or applied fields. In these meetings, you are called upon to defend your ideas—your assertions, the evidence put forward, the purpose for your work—and to convince those present of the soundness and potential contributions of the inquiry. After all, this committee can turn you down, disapproving what you propose! The need to convince takes on higher stakes when submitting a proposal to a funding agency. The stakes here are perhaps more clear: The agency can fund, not fund, or ask for revisions—hence, the need to convince your readers of the plausibility and worth of your inquiry project.

Next, some clarification of terms:

- An *argument* is generally a statement (or set of statements) whose purpose is to persuade or convince;
- An argument makes a central *claim* or *thesis*—the statement of a position or an assertion about some set of circumstances;

- An argument depends on *evidence* that the reader finds credible, that is, sufficient to support the claims made;

- The argument and its supporting evidence are made explicit through *warrants*, which bridge the gap between the evidence and the claim or assertion, providing reasoning that shows the relevance of the evidence to the claim; and

- A strong argument *acknowledges and responds* to other, perhaps disputative, views.

These ideas are summarized well by Booth, Colomb, and Williams (2008) in a book chapter entitled "Argument as a Conversation with Readers." Their remarks are made in the context of writing research reports, an activity central to graduate school. They note:

> In a research report, you make a *claim*, back it with *reasons*, support them with *evidence*, acknowledge and *respond* to other views, and sometimes explain your *principles* of reasoning. (p. 108)

Note the use of the metaphor of "conversation." This leads quite directly into consideration of the audience: Who are your readers? Your conversational partners? To whom are you addressing your written work? Who needs to be convinced of the soundness and credibility of the argument? Considering audience and purpose are central to developing sound arguments. We provide examples from everyday life to help clarify these important elements of building strong arguments (see Learning Activities 5.1–5.4 at the end of this chapter).

ENTERING THE CONVERSATION: YOUR COMMUNITY OF PRACTICE

Building a conceptual framework is complicated and messy. Students often ask how to begin. A convincing argument must be grounded in the literature (research, theories, policies, reports of practice); specifically, it must be supported by theoretical constructs that help to illuminate the topic. This is where students sometimes get stuck. We suggest that they begin with their personal insights, discuss these with their community of practice, and then turn to searching in the literature. However, this process is often reversed: Students have read in their field and come with ideas, theories, and knowledge of previous research, which then need to be critically examined through and with their community of practice. This refinement—and quite often new insights—is essential for a relatively economical search through reams and reams of potentially relevant research and appropriate theories. For example, Reilly recognizes that a lot is known about any topic at hand, but he tends to categorize the known as unitary, one body: "*This* is the lit you need to look at." Dialogue with his peers exposes the limitations of his categorization and opens up other possibilities: What does Reilly mean by neoliberalism? How—and where and when—do others use it? Where does it come from? How is it applied to specific events, activities, and people? Eventually, he sees that his label encompasses multiple interpretations and that other perspectives may be equally illuminating.

> Community of practice = your face-to-face colleagues and critical friends.

Alternatively, Kevin's interests stem from his individual professional experience as a high school principal. He has not thought about research that may expand his views. His community of practice can help him recognize that several differing and alternative literatures apply to the role of the principal and eventually help him raise new questions that mean more to him than the general ideas he held. Specifically, his peers' questions led him to uncover his deep concerns for adolescent boys, the lack of role models, and potential roles for principals. They helped Kevin find his passion and connect it with existing literature.

Again, as suggested earlier, we find it useful to use the metaphor of "conversations" when thinking about creating conceptual frameworks. You enter into conversations and shape and mold them as you develop the core ideas. These conversations have many participants: yourself with your passion and interests; peers and professors who help you craft a solid perspective; and others who have written about the focus of your project. These conversational partners make up both a *community of practice* (Lave & Wenger, 1991) and a *community of discourse* (Nystrand, 1982), as discussed in Chapter 3. Central to building a strong conceptual framework is getting in touch with your passion, or *engagement*, as we have noted before. Conversations in your community of practice can help you ground this passion within a larger context of what is known and what might be learned.

ENTERING THE CONVERSATION:
YOUR ENGAGEMENT

In Chapter 1—and revisited earlier here—we emphasized the importance of your personal interests in a topic or focus for the inquiry project. Together with an intuitive understanding of some of your fundamental assumptions (see Chapter 2) and your in-depth reading of the literature, these form your perspective.

> Where does your passion lie?

But how do you identify your perspective? This usually begins with an intuitive locating: You come to the inquiry with some interests. Your head is not empty, nor are you a blank slate. These interests may be grounded in personal, sometimes quite intimate, experiences. Or they may be professional, arising from experiences you have had in your work. Or they may be scholarly, coming from intriguing theories or research you have read. To complicate matters more, your initial interests in the topic may be some complex mix of all of these. As Schram (2006) notes, this initial intuitive locating "represent[s] a complex mix of direct experience, professional insight, intellectual orientation, intuition, emotional investment, and common sense" (p. 21). Rossman recalls a graduate student in counseling psychology who wanted to focus her inquiry on the processes of healing among mothers who had lost children. The student herself had lost children when they were quite young—her personal interests in this inquiry were deep and abiding. But she was also pursuing certification as a counselor and hoped to build a practice that would, in part, serve mothers in the processes of grieving and healing. To build a conceptual framework, her challenge was to link these personal–professional interests to scholarly work that was relevant and would provide a generative framework for her inquiry.

Rallis worked with a doctoral student in sports psychology who had been a basketball player and whose profession now was coaching. While playing basketball, she had the good fortune to try out for the women's Olympic team. Although she failed to qualify for the final team, the experience changed her life. Because of her passion, she chose to focus her inquiry on the experiences of women who pursued the goal of Olympic competition with incredible single-minded purpose and actually competed in the event. She used Bloom's theory of talent development (see Bloom, 1985) to guide her exploration. Thus, her interests arose primarily from her own experience, which she linked to broader and explanatory Theory.

As depicted in the dialogue that opens this chapter, one of our characters, Martina, had lived and experienced the devastation of HIV/AIDS in her home village in Kenya. She came to graduate school with a passion for pursuing a project that might help ameliorate the painfully challenging circumstances of children affected by HIV/AIDS: specifically, orphans and children who headed households as a result of the loss of their parents. Thus, her passion and locating the focus of her project came from deeply personal experience and emotional investment. However, as a nonformal educator and as a student pursuing a doctorate in international development education, she imagined creating programs that would serve these children and might help to improve their life circumstances. As with the two other students just discussed, Martina's challenge was to link these interests—her passionate dedication to the children—to relevant scholarly work about the intersection of poverty, livelihood opportunities, and HIV/AIDS. In the process she gravitated to and eventually drew on Freirean theories about social change, oppression, and education. What drove her inquiry was her bedrock commitment to the children.

As a contrasting example, another of our characters in the dialogue, Reilly, came to graduate school with a deep commitment to student activism and with the political position that universities exploited students. His experiences in his previous two master's degree programs had exposed him to strands of neoliberal theorizing, which center on a critique of universities as becoming increasingly corporatized. Thus, what drove his inquiry project was a set of theoretical and political ideas and propositions that he was determined to "prove." His interests and passion arose from these ideas, as applied to the student organizing work that he had been engaged with during his academic career. His challenge was to interrogate these ideas with an open mind. The first step for all of these students in moving forward was to connect with their deep and sustaining interests. In locating your own focus of inquiry, it is important to get in touch with where your passion lies.

Why is engagement or even passion important? Inquiry projects sometimes take years to complete. Once apparently completed, moreover, they may well turn into long-term projects. In the short term, however, imagine the hard work of creating a conceptual framework, posing intriguing research questions, then implementing the project (with all of its unanticipated challenges and rewards), and writing it all up. What will sustain this work? Our experience has shown that students who care deeply about the focus of their projects are more likely to end up with fascinating stories to tell (formally, we call these theses or dissertations). Those who take on a project because it is convenient, because it is their professor's research agenda, or because it seems easy produce impoverished work.

But we hear you asking: Doesn't passion mean bias? This is tricky. Yes, we all have biases, but what matters in our inquiry is how we handle our biases: Do we acknowledge them? Do we recognize limitations imposed by our biases? Are we open to alternative views? In the prior examples, each of the students brought personal interest or bias, which they drew on to make their arguments and deepen their inquiry. While all four were deeply interested in the experiences of people—they wanted to understand what happened to the people in specific circumstances—they did not have a stake in the results. The fourth, however, had an explicit agenda and was certainly passionate about it, but more inclined to seek "proof" for that agenda. This is important: All but Reilly were open-minded about what they might learn. Biases come with our passions, but bias can raise an ugly head when the inquirer appears to have all the answers before beginning the project, as, it could be argued, was the case with Reilly. One question we like to ask in dissertation defenses is: What have you learned that you didn't already know? If the answer is a halting, "Well, not much," then we become worried that the person's bias has directed and limited the exploration.

ENTERING THE CONVERSATION: THE COMMUNITIES OF DISCOURSE

The conversation must, ultimately, also include those who have written about your topic—the communities of discourse. Although you do not have immediate, face-to-face conversations with these scholars (for the most part), you engage with their ideas, their assertions, the claims that they make about the topic.

As we have discussed, the relevant literature that provides the circles in the Venn diagram of your conceptual framework can include Theory, theories, scholarly research, policy statements, and reports of professional practice. Theory (with a capital *T*) is often seen as the most prestigious in many fields; in fact, a discussion of Theory is required for many such inquiry projects. As part of your

> Community of discourse = scholars, policymakers, practitioners.

socialization into graduate study and scholarship, you will learn the norms that guide scholarly research in your field. This is important! There is not one approach (more Theory, less policy; more Policy, less theory) that is the best; it depends on the professional norms within a discipline.

The discussion of relevant literature is often described as a "review of the literature," as if there were one modality and organization for this discussion. Such is not the case. Lively, engaging, even original discussions of relevant writings of other authors are not formulaic, nor should they be tedious to read. We caution students that this creative, integrative writing is *not* the mere recitation or listing of "so-and-so found this; such-and-such found that"—what we describe as "annotated bibliographies." The process of reading, reviewing, finding links to other authors and key works, critiquing them, and locating counterdiscussions, along with all the hard intellectual work associated with these activities is frustrating, engaging, challenging, and ultimately rewarding.

Recall the discussion of models of creativity in Chapter 3. We drew from the work of Bargar and Duncan (1982), who specifically wrote about encouraging creative work at the doctoral level. The tasks of reading, reviewing, and finding links to other works maps neatly onto the *immersion* phase of the creative process. You immerse yourself in ideas, assertions, findings from research, claims—these foment in your preconscious mind, percolating away during the *incubation* phase. These two phases can be the most frustrating because overall logic and organization have not yet emerged for how *you* want to represent your fundamental argument: its central assertions, the evidence you will bring forward, links between evidence and claims, and so on. We often remind students of this, cautioning that they must allow time and space for this incubation to take place. We also provide deadlines for those who get stuck in incubation.

> A review of the literature is *not* an annotated bibliography.

Our experience suggests that insight, or illumination, follows—the "aha" experience—which indicates that an organizing schema has emerged. This, then, may well become the map for the conceptual framework. However, another cautionary note: There is tedious, painstaking work ahead, what Bargar and Duncan call "verification" (1982, p. 5). Another term for this that we use is "development." Both terms capture the hard work of filling in the assertions, claims, and evidence that flesh out the framework and its central arguments. In following this process, especially allowing ideas, readings, and Theories to incubate and attending to your insights, you claim your intellectual space.

Reading and reviewing relevant literature is often challenging because there are few simple strategies; it is sometimes tedious work. Students may well think of a literature review as a list of publications relevant to their topic; as a survey of what is out there; or, as we noted earlier, as an annotated bibliography. None of these captures the richness and generativity of a well-developed review of what others have written. At best, a review of the literature helps you to:

- *Learn* what is known about the topic and where the gaps lie;
- *Learn and explain* how knowledge in the field has been developed over time;
- *Demonstrate* that you understand the linkages between the currents of thought in the field;
- *Argue* that the research you are proposing is likely to be worthwhile;
- *Explain* how the research is justified; and
- *Identify* how the research may well make a contribution to the field.

"The literature" is a vague and ambiguous term, implying a wholeness and boundedness to that literature that doesn't exist. Although this makes identifying and reviewing relevant written work challenging, we hope we have made clear that the metaphor of "conversation" helps. We see literature reviews as conversations that you enter into; you converse with:

- Scholarly traditions;
- Recognized experts;
- Empirical research;
- Experience; and
- Professional wisdom.

In the critical discussion of these writings, the literature review should:

- *Reveal* underlying assumptions behind research questions;
- *Demonstrate* that the researcher is knowledgeable about research traditions appropriate for the discipline and topic;

- *Identify* gaps—spaces where the current inquiry project can contribute; and

- *Provide* the logical groundwork for articulating and refining research questions.

At this point, some strategies for organizing your thinking about "the literature" may be helpful.

WAYS OF ORGANIZING

So far, we have explored what the literature review should accomplish and how you make sense of all you read. Now you are ready to organize the ideas and begin writing. To augment the discussion of purposes mentioned previously, Cooper (1988) describes several ways of approaching the task of putting it all together. He suggests considering the audience, focus, specific goals, authorial perspective or stance, coverage, and organization. Each is useful in working your way through the writing up of what you have learned in conversation with the communities of discourse. What is important is that the review is not an annotated bibliography, a simple list of what you have read. Rather, the review reveals that you recognize the relevant currents of thought, how they are connected, and what gaps exist. Remember that a fundamental purpose is to support the argument you have constructed and to help situate that argument within a larger context.

> Audience, audience, audience—to whom are you writing?

Thinking about your *audience* is a fundamental step. Since you are in graduate school, the most likely audience for a literature review is a scholarly one: your advisors and examiners and other scholars in the field. Your review, critique, analysis, and synthesis of the literature should, therefore, keep this audience firmly in mind; you should speak to this audience. This suggests a *focus* on relevant theory/ies, research findings or outcomes, and perhaps research methods. A scholarly audience wants to be convinced that you know and understand the key theories and research studies conducted that are relevant for your topic. However, in applied fields, such as education, public health, public policy, or management, a focus on applications for practice may also be appropriate and quite useful. Thus, your review should address theories and research, but it may emphasize the implications for, let's say, management of not-for-profit small businesses. As another example, Rallis and her coauthors began their how-to book for school principals with a practitioner-oriented chapter reviewing and critiquing what is already known about principal leadership (Militello, Rallis, & Goldring, 2009).

The relative emphasis within the review is also shaped by your *specific goals,* which may be:

- *To offer an integrative discussion,* which could include developing generalizations across research findings, resolving conflicting per- spectives or research findings, and/or building connections across key ideas or concepts articulated in theories;
- *To critique the existing literature,* identifying shortcomings (perhaps historical) or inadequate analyses;
- *To identify central issues* or questions that will frame your inquiry project; and
- *To identify gaps* where your project will contribute.

As you write, you embody your *authorial perspective,* or *stance,* relative to the topic and the discourses that you converse with. We have discussed the centrality of your perspective throughout; in writing, you articulate this perspective and build the central argument that frames your project. His- torically and, in some disciplines, to the present, this notion of authorial perspective is anathema. With epistemological assumptions that are more objectivist (see Chapter 2), the norms in these disciplines stipulate an appar- ently neutral authorial stance. Recall the discussion about James Watson and Barbara McClintock, Nobel laureates whose open espousal of their very deep—and very personal—engagement with their topics was present in their bodies of work. Both use the first person throughout their work. As before, we caution you to consider your audience and the prevailing norms of the relevant communities of practice and discourse.

Finally, the *coverage* and *organization* of a literature review are cru- cial for developing your overall argument and framework. Again, histori- cally, literature reviews were supposed to be "exhaustive" (and, as we note, exhausting!). In some fields and with some topics, this may be possible, but many inquiry projects represent the intersection of currents of thought: the overlapping circles in a Venn diagram. You need to become immersed in the relevant theories and research about your topic, but we encourage students to lift the burden of having this immersion be exhaustive. Rather, consider that the discussion of relevant literature can focus on authors and/ or works that are "representative" or "central" or "pivotal." This will entail learning which authors and key pieces of scholarly work are, in fact, representative or central, but articulating that your review will be one or the other helps the audience understand the scope and boundaries you have placed around it.

How you *organize* the review is often where you demonstrate creativity, new insights, and certainly the overall framework. Simply categorizing by the currents of thought you followed will not reveal your analyses and syntheses of what you read. Consider arranging your review in any of the following ways: historical or chronological, conceptual or thematic, pivotal moments, or methodological (i.e., by the various methods used by researchers on the problem or issue). Obviously, an overall historical organization could include a focus on methodology within key time periods in the development of thought within the field; thus, creative blending of these structures of organization is always possible.

With these ideas in mind, you have some "hooks" to help guide you through the processes of reading and critiquing and writing about the literature that is the core of your conceptual framework. As you engage in this work, keep in mind that you are developing *your* intellectual stance that will guide your inquiry project.

This chapter has focused on the complex processes of developing a conceptual framework for an inquiry project. As we noted at the beginning, this is very much an iterative process as you examine your own interests for an intuitive locating of the project; delve into theories, research, policy statements, reports of practice on the topic—the currents of thought; revisit your intuitive framing; read more literature; and so on. Note that the preliminary framework you are constructing will also be refined and shaped as you consider *how* you will implement the project; we discuss these important considerations in Chapter 6. We close this chapter by emphasizing how important a clear conceptual framework is for any inquiry project: for providing direction, for raising intriguing research questions, and for foreshadowing the design. In summary, your conceptual framework reveals the route of your journey.

Learning Activity 5.1. One Study, Four Representations

To engage you in the need for building a convincing argument, we invite you to review four versions of essentially the same ideas: research on IQ and birth order. Our purpose is to encourage critical thinking about audience and who might be convinced by each representation and central argument.

In our classes we provide four quite different versions of a study on IQ and birth order. You could use our example or find any four perspectives on some idea. We selected the particular research about birth order based on the assumption that each of you is part of a family and therefore may well be interested in the study. The versions come from the following sources:

> The journal *Science, 316*(22) (2007), downloaded from *www.sciencemag.org*

> A news report on the study published in the *New York Times* (*www.nytimes.com/2007/06/21/science/21cnd-sibling. html?hp=&pagewanted=print*)

> A commentary on the study in the June 2007 *Slate* magazine (*www. Slate.com*)

> An interactive blog on the study, also found on the *Slate* website

Once you have read the different reports and commentaries, we invite you to think about and discuss with your critical friends which version of the study seems the most "true," "correct," or "credible." Be careful not to assume that the report in *Science* is/must be the most authoritative because it is a research report.

One outcome we hope for is that you will begin to understand that formal "research reports" are only one representation of knowledge, one that society tends to valorize. Most of us think, "It's a research report, so it must be true!" The discussions focus on purpose and audience, important concepts to integrate into your thinking. The conversation also focuses on how different representations are, or are not, "legitimate," as discussed in Chapter 3, in terms of norms of scholarship. This, in turn, invites introspection about your personal inquiry perspective.

Questions we ask:

- What is the fundamental argument? The major point?
- What is the central claim or assertion?

- What is put forward as evidence?
- What evidence seems most valid (to you), and why?
- What is the purpose of each different article? Who is the intended audience?
- Which representation has the most credibility (to/for you)?

Learning Activity 5.2. Developing a Position

Writing memos helps you articulate what you are interested in—the focus of a possible inquiry project—and helps you develop a set of assertions around your perspective on the topic. Three related memoing exercises are described next.

Guidelines

This first assignment asks you to choose an issue or topic that is important to you. Because our field is education, we ask you to make an assertion or a set of related assertions (something they believe to be true) about a type of educational organization (e.g., schools, universities, nonformal programs) or process (e.g., policymaking, decision making, learning). Your assertion can be related to the field in which you are studying. You should define key terms and explain how you *know* that your assertion has merit or why you believe it to be true. Put simply, you identify your standpoint and how that shapes the assertion. We ask: Where are you coming from? What experience or knowledge shapes your assertion? What assumptions have you made that support this assertion? To develop skills of writing concisely, we ask that the paper be no more than two pages.

Group Discussion

Work together in your critical inquiry triads (see Learning Activity 3.2) or in another relevant group to critique each other's position papers. Questions to guide this dialogue are clarifying questions only. Our expectation here is that you will help one another get more clear about what each person believes to be true (their knowledge), how their experience is shaping their knowledge claims (their perspective), and what has led them to believe that their assertion is true (what they rely on as evidence). Next, we ask you to complicate their assertions in a second paper, described next.

Learning Activity 5.3. Complicating Your Position

Guidelines

Drawing on the first position paper and its assertions, take a different point of view that complicates the first paper. Because positions are often firmly held, we ask you to consider what someone who disagrees with this position would argue. What points would that person make? How would that person try to convince you of his or her position? This mental debate will offer a new and, it is hoped, a more complex, nuanced assertion based on that perspective. In the second memo, consider: What are your new assumptions and how do they differ from your previous ones? Finally, comment on how the new perspective has changed how you view the organization or process.

Debrief

Once again, return to your critical inquiry triads and pose questions about how the argument is developing. Focusing on assertions and counterassertions helps you understand the elements of strong argumentation. We then ask students to depict ideas primarily nonverbally through concept maps.

Learning Activity 5.4. Concept Mapping

Guidelines

We invite you to draw on the analyses in papers 1 and 2, focusing your topics a bit more and building a framework around the ideas. We suggest that you, quite literally, use bubbles and arrows and question marks to create a map of your thinking. In doing so, we suggest that you consider the following: What questions do you have about your topic now? What are the central concepts that you have been writing about? How do you think these concepts relate to one another? What currents of thought might they link to? As before, you might turn to your critical inquiry group to share and critique each other's maps: Does the map make sense? Are the connections between ideas apparent and reasonable? What is missing?

FOR FURTHER READING

→ Boote, D. N., & Beile, P. (2005). Scholars before researchers: On the centrality of the dissertation literature review in research preparation. *Educational Researcher, 34*(6), 3–15.

→ Cooper, H. (2009). *Research synthesis and meta-analysis* (4th ed.). Thousand Oaks, CA: Sage.

→ Fink, A. (2010). *Conducting research literature reviews: From the Internet to paper* (3rd ed.). Thousand Oaks, CA: Sage.

→ Hart, C. (2002). *Doing a literature review: Releasing the social science research imagination*. London: Sage.

→ Ling, P. M. (2008). *Preparing literature reviews: Qualitative and quantitative approaches* (3rd ed.). Glendale, CA: Pyrczak.

→ Schram, T. H. (2006). *Conceptualizing and proposing qualitative research* (2nd ed.). Upper Saddle River, NJ: Pearson Merrill Prentice Hall.

→ Schratz, M., & Walker, R. (1995). *Research as social change: New opportunities for qualitative research*. London: Routledge. See Chapter 6: "Theory Is Not Just Theoretical."

Designing the Inquiry Project

Finding "True North"

⊛ *Critical Questions to Guide Your Reading*

↪ *What are various options for design and research methods? (remembering)*

↪ *What are the unique features of each option? (understanding)*

↪ *What is the relationship between designs and methods? (analyzing)*

↪ *How would various designs and methods apply to my inquiry project? (applying)*

↪ *Which options might be most generative for my work? (evaluating)*

↪ *How might I design my inquiry project? (creating)*

Dialogue 6. Considering Design Options

Professor Bettara opened the class by calling on three volunteers to share with the rest of the class their very preliminary ideas about how they're actually going to implement their projects; this is more formally called "design." The student volunteers were somewhat anxious about these more public walk-throughs because they had, up to now, shared their ideas only in their triads (and with the professor). Now, they would share them with the whole class. They weren't sure whether the trust they felt in their triads (for the most part) would obtain with everyone listening to them! After reassuring them privately, Bettara began class by outlining key principles for the exercise. First, the volunteers each had about 10 minutes to share their ideas; after this, other class members could raise questions or make comments. These questions or comments, however, had to be in the spirit of being good critical friends, as they had all practiced in their triads. Bettara reminded the volunteers that they only had to listen to and consider the questions or comments of their classmates; in fact, they did not need to respond. The class began with Samira.

SAMIRA: Well, I'm a bit nervous about this, but here goes. My triad partners know that I'm very interested in why students of color just don't make it in college. To me, it's a social justice issue. Why should black or brown students have such trouble? What are colleges doing to help them out? What *aren't* they doing?

Some ideas I've thought about. (*Turns to use the chalkboard.*) First, I could do a survey of students of color in a couple of colleges, just to find out what their attitudes are and maybe something about their backgrounds. I think I've seen this sort of study done, but I have some concerns. It's like continuing to "blame the victim." Just finding out more about them means that the fix needs to be in them. Well, that's one.

Two, I could analyze student support programs to find out what they are doing for students of color. But again, it might be the same problem of blaming the students, though indirectly. Do you know what I mean? (*Nods.*) Or should I do something that really involves them, like a PAR [participatory action research] project with a small group of students at one campus—maybe even here— to help them look critically at their situations? Very Freirean, but very time consuming. I'm also concerned about taking up too much of *their* time. Would that be ethical? But would it be ethical *not* to involve them? This way might make more of a difference in the long run, if the students decided to take some action, but there are so many challenges. And they might even believe that no one will listen to them—like, when was the last time the president here paid attention to students?!! So, I'm just not sure which way to go. Any ideas?

MARTINA: Samira, can you talk a little bit more about what you want to learn? That might help us to help you better. Remember that chapter from Knight [2002, Ch. 2] about the claims you want to make at the end? What might you learn that could make a difference for the students?

SAMIRA: Good questions. I'll have to think about them. Sometimes it just seems too overwhelming. And I'm really worried about the sample. . . . Others?

KEVIN: Wow, Samira. It's like my concerns about the boys in my school and what I can learn that will make a difference for them. What about doing something that both surveys and interviews people? Would that make sense?

RAUL: Would that be too much to tackle? Doing surveys right is not easy, and interviews, transcribing and all, takes a lot of time.

REILLY: No, I think you should do an ethnography, a critical ethnography. After all, your questions are all about power, justice, who gets what, who doesn't, why. Think about new institutional theory here. You know, what DiMaggio and Powell [1991] write about. Don't they use ethnographic methods? Yeah, do an ethnography of a college that's got a really bad track record with students of color. How about that?

RAUL: Or maybe a really good track record. Or both and analyze what's different and similar.

MARTINA: I just realized that I'm not sure what you really want to accomplish. Like, what's your purpose?

SAMIRA: Wow! Thanks, you guys. There are some really good ideas here, but how do I choose? Now I need to just think about these for a while. And I've got to think about other things, like where I can do this and what it will take. You know . . . feasibility. But thanks.

Bettara had been writing the comments and questions on the chalkboard and asked if there were any more. Samira was then invited to consider these ideas as she moved more deeply into designing an ethical, do-able inquiry project.

Clearly, Samira and her classmates have moved along in conceptualizing their inquiry projects; they have a clearer idea of *what* they want to learn. Now, their challenge is to consider *how* they are going to learn; they begin to design their studies. Before we discuss the elements to weigh and ponder in designing a study, we want to recall the conundrum mentioned in Chapter 5. That conundrum was as follows: To enter into a detailed exploration of the literature, you need a preliminary conceptual framework as a guide. However, you will find it difficult to begin to develop such a framework without some understanding of the relevant literature. To deal with this conundrum, we recommend that you delve into the literature, step back and do some hard thinking (conceptualizing), and then reenter the literature with a better sense of a roadmap.

We take a similar position about two other important linkages: the relationship between the conceptual framework and the design (the *what* and the *how*) and, within the latter, the relationship between the overall design and specific research methods. To explicate, you start with *what* and move to your *how* (design), which, in turn, may modify your *what*. We assert that

> The *how* emerges from the *what*.

conceptualizing an inquiry project should *not* be driven by the research design and especially not by methods. Although weighing the feasibility of particular designs and methods is crucial, your ultimate decisions should logically and organically flow from the framework and the research questions. Similarly, determining the overall design of a study is difficult, if not impossible, without some sense of appropriate research methods. However, to repeat, the overall logic and approach to a study should *not* be driven by methods; it should be driven by the conceptual framework and research questions. You can't plan your itinerary if you don't know where you're headed (e.g., if you want an action–adventure vacation, you are not likely to choose a secluded yoga retreat). With too much focus on methods, the danger arises that the methods will drive the research questions that are addressed rather than the other way around. We are deeply concerned about the student who, when asked what his or her research project is about, says "Oh, I'm doing a survey." In such cases, the methods are driving the design; the resulting study may well be limited in value unless it is grounded in a well-thought-out conceptual framework.

We have noted that several research texts discuss specific methods first and then move into a discussion of research design. As one example, Knight

(2002) presents "Face-to-Face Inquiry Methods" (Chapter 3—observation, interviews, focus groups) and "Research at a Distance" (Chapter 4—questionnaires, attitude measures). He then follows these with a chapter on research design. This is typical of many research texts. Although we recognize the merit of this organization, it may well encourage students to land on a particular method (one that seems felicitous or even easy) and then figure out a design that will allow them to use this method. By the same logic, students can fixate on a particular method, revising the conceptual framework and research questions to suit that method. Although the process is, in reality, iterative—that is, as you consider designs and methods, you refine your conceptual framework, particularly the research questions—you must have a start point: the conceptual framework, *not* the methods or design. Possible choices about methods (or design) must be critically examined in light of the conceptual framework. Up to now, you have developed an argument, reviewed the literature, identified gaps, and raised questions. Now you are choosing a way to inform the questions. The questions, in practice, provide the bridge between the conceptual framework and the design.

MOVING FROM THE CONCEPTUAL FRAMEWORK INTO DESIGN

Recall from Chapter 5 that one of the purposes of the conceptual framework with its review of relevant literatures is to identify gaps in what is known. The discussion of literature—empirical research on the topic, appropriate and generative theories and concepts, policy statements, evaluations of practice—should support your central argument that Problem X can be usefully explored by drawing on Y and Z currents of thought. However, you have identified gaps in what is known: unanswered questions, tensions and disagreements, proposed solutions that need to be tested further. In building this argument, you accomplish at least four things:

1. You *connect* your proposed inquiry to the ongoing discourses in your field;
2. You *show* how your inquiry will contribute to those discourses;
3. You *demonstrate* what is known and what is *not* known; and
4. You *argue* that your inquiry will help to fill that gap.

In building this argument, you articulate the purpose for your inquiry and stipulate the research questions that will guide it. Purpose and research questions are crucial; they are the anchor points to which you will return again and again to keep you on course. They serve as your "true North."

Determining Purpose

Establishing purpose is central to your entire inquiry project. The purpose is your goal, your aim, your guide, your intention—*what* you want to accomplish though your inquiry project. As mentioned, purpose serves as your "true North"—where you are heading. It keeps you on track through all the exciting but often distracting side roads that any inquiry project goes through. Establishing your purpose helps you to be crystal clear about the research questions that will frame and provide further direction for your project. Establishing purpose is essential for the design of the study.

What are useful purposes for inquiry projects? Throughout the historic literature on research methods, four purposes are most frequently mentioned:

1. To *describe*—to summarize, gather information, or map elements of, for example, social interactions in the workplace, a historical period, beliefs about presidential candidates, actions of waves on shorelines;

2. To *explore*—to discover, generate, uncover new information; to identify similarities or differences;

3. To *explain*—to identify reasons for, understand connections and relationships, test why phenomena occur in particular ways, compare cases of phenomena; and

4. To *predict*—to forecast, with reasonable confidence, what will happen in a particular situation.

These are the four canonical purposes for research. However, we would add that, with more critical perspectives on inquiry, an additional primary purpose could also be (Rossman & Rallis, 2012, p. 129):

5. To *empower*—to foster, encourage a sense of agency with groups and individuals. (We note that often empowerment is accomplished through description, exploration, explanation, or prediction.)

Note that all purposes are stated as verbs that imply an action. Synonyms, such as *test* or *compare*, for these canonical purposes are useful to play with, as you are developing your purpose. A simplified grouping of purposes that you might find helpful is to describe, to compare or relate, or to test or predict.

Grappling with your purpose is an essential but often frustrating exercise because purposes can overlap and become conflated with one another. However, we argue that *description* is foundational to all other purposes; that is, you cannot *explore* new areas, *explain* complex phenomena, or *predict* what may happen without a solid grounding in description. To complicate matters, our position is that description is never merely description; there is always analysis and, quite often, explanation or interpretation that attends a project even if its purpose is stated as "description." To explore a phenomenon, you have to describe it. Further, you must know what the phenomenon is like (description) before you can explain why it is the way it is or before you can make justified predictions. To us, then, description is the bedrock; what you decide to do beyond that is captured in your purpose statements and the research questions, to which we now turn.

Stipulating Research Questions

Settling on generative, succinct, and useful research questions takes time and much revising, imagining how they would work, and informally trying them out. This is often best done with a community of practice—those trusted individuals who can gently challenge you and offer suggestions. In general, research questions call for analytic descriptions, seek to discover or establish a relationship, or propose to test a hypothesis.

Research questions are typically broad questions that set the general direction and provide focus for the inquiry. These are often called "grand tour" (Rossman & Rallis, 2012, p. 132). These broad questions are then followed by a parsimonious number of subquestions, which can fruitfully be thought of as implementing questions. Given the specific choice of the design and methods, formal hypotheses may then be cast. The research questions should be critically examined by asking the following:

- Does this question flow directly from the conceptual framework?
- Is the logical development from the literature to this question clear?
- Does this question implement my purpose?

- Is this question important? Will it help advance knowledge in my field?
- Am I interested in the question? Will pursuing this question engage me sufficiently throughout the project?
- What are the potential ethical challenges I may encounter in addressing this question?
- Can I gather data (or do data already exist) that will help me to respond to this question?

These questions can be summarized in three key criteria for conducting any inquiry (Rossman & Rallis, 2012, pp. 114–118; see Figure 6.1):

1. The study is *do-able*. It is feasible in terms of sufficient resources (my, and others', time and energy; money; knowledge and skills; support);

2. The study is *want-to-do-able*: I have the passion, engagement, and commitment to carry the project through to completion; and

3. The study is *should-do-able*: The ethical issues that I foresee do not seem to be overwhelming, the study is likely to contribute to advancing knowledge in my field, and the study has the potential to help improve the human condition.

We now move into an extended example of Samira's nascent inquiry project, as touched on in the dialogue that began this chapter. Samira is at the point where considering different purposes and research questions—

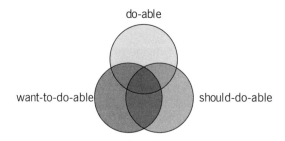

FIGURE 6.1. Considerations in design. From Rossman and Rallis (2012, p. 115). Copyright 2012 by Sage Publications, Inc. Reprinted by permission.

trying them on, if you will—helps her to land in a place where her interests and passions are fully engaged. Thus, we recommend several walk-throughs to help focus and determine purpose. The process is complex and iterative, but it can be energizing and fruitful.

Samira's interest arises from her concerns about social justice and equity in colleges and universities. She cares deeply about students of color and is concerned that the retention and graduation rates of these students are well below those of white middle-class students. Given these commitments, Samira begins to consider different purposes for her project.

Focusing on *description* (and by this we mean analytic description), Samira might stipulate the following overall research questions:

- *What* are the characteristics of students who graduate from college?
- *What* are the characteristics of students who drop out of college?

Before you criticize these questions too sharply, recall that Samira is at the beginning of a process: Should she stay with this primary purpose and line of questioning, she will develop implementing questions, and she will go on to consider various research designs and methods, as discussed shortly.

Should Samira be interested in an *exploratory* project, she might ask "What aspects of college students' experiences support retention?" To pursue this purpose, she would have to demonstrate, through the literature review, that there are few empirical studies on this topic. She is then justified in claiming that she is exploring a little-studied phenomenon. An *explanatory* purpose might lead her to ask, "Why do certain aspects of the college students' experiences support retention?" Note the shift here to *why*; previous questions have begun with *what*. The *why* question signals a quest for explanation, whereas *what* questions invite analytic description. With this question, she would be interested in analyzing various aspects of experiences to determine which were closely associated with patterns of retention. A *predictive* purpose could be addressed through a question such as "Do students from professional-class backgrounds graduate at higher rates than those from the working classes?" She would, of course, have to elaborate the "yes" or "no" response that this question implies. With answers to this question, Samira would then be able to predict, based on socioeconomic status, what percentage of an entering cohort of first-year students is likely to graduate. Within this predictive purpose, Samira may embed a hypothesis that emerges from her reading: "Students of color who come from professional-class backgrounds graduate at higher rates than students of color from working-class backgrounds."

However, given Samira's grounding in social justice and equity issues, she might want to focus her project on one with *empowerment* as its overall purpose. While she is mindful that she herself cannot empower others, she might be able to create a set of experiences that encourage a sense of agency among the students she works with. This is an explicitly egalitarian and action research–oriented approach; thus, her grand tour question might be: "Does engaging students in critical assessment of their experiences encourage them to stay in college?"

As noted, there are useful synonyms and refining terms for thinking about purpose. Should Samira want to explicitly *relate* two variables, she might ask, "Does grade point average relate to retention?" Or she might want to *test* the question, "Does X program increase graduation rates?" (through processes of randomization, discussed in greater detail later).

Along with her community of practice, Samira now moves into considering just what the *how* of the study might be. With some idea about possible purposes and research questions (at least the big ones), she can turn to thinking about the overall design for her project. Again, we hope that she will weigh various alternatives in light of her possible purpose and research questions *and* possible methods. Next, we walk you—and Samira—through some typical research designs. Our purpose here is to engage you in thinking about the array of ways to approach an inquiry project. Where you finally settle will be the result of a complex mix of the prevailing norms in your discipline, your interests, your methodological training, and the feasibility of the various options—not easy, but giving this process sufficient time yields a tighter, more well-thought-through proposal.

CONSIDERING VARIOUS DESIGNS

In our teaching, we have found it useful to expose students to a variety of designs for implementing their inquiry projects. We do this because all too often students conflate research methods with design. Such is not the case, although some designs *do* stipulate specific methods. For our students, we provide short descriptions of what each design is typically intended to accomplish (back to purpose) and some examples, and we provide a handful here (see also Table 6.1). This is, of necessity, a brief introduction to research designs; this limited overview assumes that you will delve into design and specific methods as you move along. Note that any of these designs can rest comfortably within a whole raft of theoretical perspectives (back to conceptual framework). We then return to the extended example of Samira's work and show options she might pursue, given the research questions she has been considering.

TABLE 6.1. Design Options		
	Typical purpose	**Typical methods**
Observation designs	To gather information on real-time behaviors, actions, and interactions	Observation protocols, open-ended ethnographic observation
In-depth interview designs	To understand individual or group perspectives, views, and feelings	Face-to-face discussions or conversations
Document analysis designs	To analyze patterns in various texts or cultural artifacts	Guided analysis and interpretation
Case study designs	In-depth study of one instance of a phenomenon	Multiple methods
Survey designs	To describe trends in a population; to identify the distribution of characteristics or frequency of attitudes or practices	Questionnaires; frequently Web based
Correlation designs	To measure the degree of association between two or more variables	Data sources may include responses to assessments, socioeconomic data, etc.
Comparative designs	To compare and contrast two or more instances of a phenomenon	Multiple methods
Action research designs	To experiment, test out, and critically reflect on practice	Multiple methods
Quasi-experimental designs	To test the relative strength of an intervention	Multiple methods
Randomized controlled trials	With more power than quasi-experimental designs, to test the relative strength of an intervention	Sampling and assignment are randomized; multiple methods

Observation Designs

The overall purpose of observational designs is to gather information on behaviors, actions, and interactions in real time. Their purposes are typically analytic description or exploration. Observations can reveal patterns or allow comparisons, but it is challenging to derive robust explanations for actions and behaviors through observation alone. To focus the attention of the inquirer, observation designs may rely on checklists or detailed observation protocols. Observational designs, however, may stipulate ethnographic observation, which generally begins with a wide-angle lens, then focuses the observations, and then may return to a wide view. Or they may be open-ended visual surveys. Such designs may generate data that are narratives of what was observed or data in the form of numbers when specific behaviors or actions are counted. This design stipulates a method for gathering data—observations—although the specific observational approach remains to be defined in the methods section.

In-Depth Interview Designs

Depending on purpose and questions, a study may also be fruitfully designed as a series of in-depth interviews. In-depth interview studies are intended to understand individual perspectives about a phenomenon. Commonly exploratory or explanatory, such studies rely on often deeply personal face-to-face "conversations." Group interviews may describe, explore, or seek to explain collective perspectives. Although such studies typically generate narratives, at times mention of specific incidents or concepts may be enumerated. This design also stipulates a method, but, again, the particular interviewing philosophy and approach will be discussed in the methods section.

Document Analysis Designs

Designs focusing on documents are intended to provide analytic description, and perhaps explanation of some phenomenon, of "cultural artifacts"—that is, existing documents. Such documents might be policy papers, newspapers, novels, and so on. The focus may be historical or contemporary expressions of culture that are signified in documents. As with the two designs just presented, such analyses may generate narratives or numbers. This design, too, stipulates the method—analysis of document; details will follow in the methods section.

Case Study Designs

Case study designs are intended to study in depth one instance of a phenomenon; in multisite case studies, there are, obviously, more "cases" that are investigated. Case studies are intended to capture complexity and context; their often open-ended nature encourages the inquirer to ask about what is not yet known or obvious. Given that, case study designs are useful for analytic description, exploration, and perhaps explanation. Cross-case analyses and interpretation allow for contrast and comparison. Case study designs do not stipulate specific methods: They typically draw on multiple methods and multiple data sources.

Survey Designs

Survey designs are intended to describe trends in a population; to identify the distribution of characteristics across a group; to identify the frequency of attitudes or practices; and perhaps to relate two or more variables (see Correlation Designs next). Thus, survey designs provide descriptions of phenomena across a large number of units. To be able to claim that one knows distributions or frequencies or trends, random sampling is necessary. Survey designs typically rely on questionnaires as the primary method, asking respondents to provide the researcher with specific information.

Correlation Designs

Correlation designs set out to measure the degree of association between two (or more) sets of variables. These variables could be attitudes or practices, demographic characteristics, responses on standardized examinations, and so on. They are typically descriptive in purpose, seeking to describe the extent to which variables covary. Data sources may include responses to tests or assessments, demographic data, and so on. Correlation designs are not well suited to providing robust explanations or for making predictions.

Comparative Designs

Comparative designs are explicitly intended to make comparisons across two or more instances of a phenomenon. This could be a multisite case study where cases are deliberately compared with one another to ascertain similarities and differences, or a comparative policy analysis could examine policies on a specific topic across several countries, again seeking similarities and differences. Again, with this design, methods remain to be detailed in that section.

Action Research Designs

Action research designs follow the pattern of the inquiry cycle discussed in Chapter 3. This entails observing what is happening, what the results are, and then problematizing those results, trying out new practices and actions, observing what happens as a result, critically examining those results, and beginning the cycle all over again. Practitioners engage in action research to improve their practice or organizational functioning. Participatory action research is more oriented toward radical change, blurs the distinction between researcher and participants, and seeks change in oppressive structures.

A NOTE ON RANDOMIZATION

Before moving to the final two designs, we comment on the power of randomization—the *sine qua non* for making robust predictions. Randomization draws on the logic of probabilities, which allows us to make predictions, within certain confidence intervals. Through randomization, we are able to make statistical inferences about the sample and the population from which it was drawn. In contrast is the logic of comparison and contrast, which encourages extending findings from one small sample to another through reasoning processes that look for similarities and differences (i.e., compare and contrast). Although this logic does not have the power of mathematical probabilities, it is still useful for many descriptive, exploratory, and explanatory designs.

Quasi-Experimental Designs

Quasi-experimental designs are comparative in nature, seeking to ascertain differences across time, across groups, or across treatments. Typically, one would see a pretest–posttest design, where an assessment is made prior to implementation of a "treatment" and then again afterward. Comparisons can also be made across groups: those who received the treatment and those who did not. However, quasi-experimental designs lack the rigor of random-ized assignment or selection.

Randomized Controlled Trials

Randomized controlled trials (RCTs) draw on the comparative logic of quasi-experimental designs with the key addition of randomization. The "units" of interest are assigned, through processes of randomization, to a specific "treatment" (e.g., a drug trial, a pedagogical approach). A control group is also randomly selected; these do not receive the treatment. Assessments are implemented, and the results of the experimental group are compared with those of the control group. Random assignment brings the power of prob-abilities to these analyses.

When considering various designs, in addition to the "abilities" depicted in Figure 6.1, also consider whether you are interested in learning broadly across a population or in depth from a smaller number and the extent to which the design should be tightly structured or more open ended. You should also consider how you want the various elements of the design to unfold over time—the ebb and flow (see Rossman & Rallis, 2012, pp. 172–173). Remember that these are decisions that you—the inquirer—are autho-rized to make.

With these possible designs in mind (and the combinations and per-mutations are practically limitless), we return to Samira to see what overall designs she might consider for each possible research question.

SAMIRA'S RESEARCH QUESTIONS AND POSSIBLE DESIGNS

Samira's potential *descriptive research questions* (recall that we mean ana-lytic description) are: "What are the characteristics of students who gradu-ate from college? What are the characteristics of students who drop out of college?" To implement these questions, Samira could usefully consider the following: in-depth interview design, case study(ies) design, document anal-ysis design, observational design, or survey design. Her choices would be influenced by such factors as available existing data, access to key individuals, her specific interests (such as breadth or depth), observability

> Breadth or depth?
> Prefigured or open-ended?
> Ebb and flow?

(i.e., can she see the characteristics?), resources (i.e., time and skills), and existence and availability of relevant documents.

Samira's *exploratory* question, "What aspects of students' college experiences support retention?", could be implemented through an in-depth interview design, survey design, document analysis design, or case study design. An observational design would not be practical for this type of question because observations might generate too much irrelevant data. As well, quasi-experimental designs or RCTs would be difficult to implement given her focus, but would provide solid answers to this question. The *explanatory* question, "Why do certain aspects of the college students' experiences support retention?", could rely on the same designs as for the exploratory question, with a different purpose.

The *predictive* question, "Do students from professional class backgrounds graduate more frequently than those from working class?", would benefit from either a comparative case study design (comparing the two groups over time) or a comparative statistical analyses design, in which the variable of socioeconomic status was tested against graduation. A second predictive question, "Does Program X increase graduation rates?", could be explored through a quasi-experimental design where students participating in Program X are compared with those not participating in the program. If Program X had an effect, Samira could predict that participation would increase graduate rates.

Finally, Samira's *empowerment question*, "Does engaging students in critical assessment of their experiences encourage retention to graduation?", would best be addressed through a case study with action research design. Note, however, the predictive connotations of this question: If Samira learns that students stay in college and graduate after participating in the critical assessment activities, she could, gently, predict that such activities hold promise for retention.

As you consider Samira's experience in weighing and seriously considering various designs, ask yourself the following questions (adapted from Schram, 2006, p. 111):

- When and how do I settle on a generative design?
- Does this design emerge logically from my conceptual framework?
- Do I have to follow a particular design formulaically, or can I adapt it to suit my needs and interests?
- How does grappling with various designs help to focus and strengthen my inquiry?

A SHORT COURSE ON RESEARCH METHODS

In this next section, we take you through a very brief discussion of some research methods. Our intent here is to expose you to these methods; additional readings on each are found at the end of this chapter. We assume that you will take courses—or engage in independent inquiry—to learn about research methods in depth sufficient to implement your inquiry project in trustworthy and robust ways. However, we have found that even this limited exposure helps trigger students' imaginations about possibilities. This helps move them from a received knowledge of what is possible to a more open imagined space. Although tedious, many students find inspiration in just knowing about the variety of methods available to them.

Questionnaires

We have all been invited to complete questionnaires. The U.S. Census is one example; you can think of many more. The purpose of questionnaires is to ask respondents a series of questions about the topic of interest. Questionnaires can be conducted via mail, telephone, or, increasingly, online through software such as SurveyMonkey®. The art of questionnaire design lies in the questions and the response categories provided. Researchers may use a validated instrument or construct their own. Creating a reliable and valid questionnaire demands considerable knowledge of psychometrics as well as precise piloting procedures. As with any method, pilot testing is crucial for determining whether the questions and response categories are useful and valid and will provide the hoped-for information.

Attitudinal/Behavioral Measures

If you were a student in a U.S. college undergraduate *Introductory Psychology* class, you more than likely were asked to respond to some sort of attitude or behavior assessment. These are similar to questionnaires, but may include items that can cross-check responses with one another. Examples include attitudes toward smoking, alcohol and drug use, nonresident immigrant populations, and so on. Behavioral assessments focus on what people report they actually do or have done rather than on their attitudes toward X. Behavioral assessments might ask if one smokes or uses drugs. Again, the art of designing such instruments lies in the questioning. When asking about particularly risky behaviors (e.g., smoking, drug use, drunk driving), ethical considerations are high, as are concerns about whether respondents are telling you what they *think* they should say—called "response bias" or "socially acceptable responses." Again, using an existing instrument may be possible; generating one's own assessment tools can be quite time consuming.

Achievement/Performance Measures

Standardized tests are well-known examples of achievement measures. Primary and secondary examinations, as well as college and graduate school admissions tests, are familiar to us all. Typically, the researcher using these sorts of measures as data will rely on existing databases: a school district's test scores, scores on the SAT available from the Educational Testing Service, and so on. Such measures can be quite useful for a comparative study.

Document and Artifact Analyses

Also an overall design, document and artifact analysis entails the researcher identifying those documents or artifacts of interest and conducting analyses of them, based on his research questions. Documents are frequently used in this method, but the researcher may also be interested in objects—the artifacts that a group or society produces: photographs, clothing, pottery, trash. Clearly, the focus and selection of documents and artifacts depend on the purpose of the inquiry and the research questions.

Interviews

An overall design and a face-to-face method, interviewing entails asking people questions and eliciting detailed responses. Many forms and strategies for interviewing exist; all, however, involve conversations with the interview partners. Interviewing can be framed by a number of theoretical perspectives and take place with a variety of different groups. Focus group interviews, which seek collective understanding, are one variation on interviewing where several (no more than about 10) are interviewed for their shared perspectives on the topic.

Observation

Also an overall design, observation as a data-gathering method means just that: sitting and attending to the actions and interactions in the setting. Observation may be structured through protocols that require the observer to note only certain actions or interactions, or they may be open ended, in which the ebb and flow of everyday life in the setting is recorded through extensive field notes.

Photos and Videos

Photographs and videos are another generative research method. The researcher records actions and interactions through a camera or video recorder, thereby creating a permanent record that can be reviewed again and again. The advantages of photographs and videos are that they include facial expressions, body movement, and other nonverbal signals. However, photos and videos are not objective representations. As a cautionary note, in today's digital age when nothing is ever fully erased from cyberspace or when digitized data can be altered, ethical considerations must be addressed.

There are many, many other research methods that can be generative for your particular inquiry project. Learning about them is exciting but can be overwhelming. Our advice is that you be sure that the choice of methods flows from your conceptual framework and research questions and fits your design. We also look for a parsimonious number of methods: too many methods, yielding too much data, can lead to analysis paralysis! Keep it simple.

PLANNING FOR ANALYSIS AND INTERPRETATION

Having chosen the research questions, design, and possible methods for collecting data to inform those questions, you should make some initial plans for making sense of the data, that is, analyzing them. What you do with the data is critically important. Discoveries and answers do not simply emerge; instead, you *construct* knowledge through a systematic reasoning process that begins when you conceptualize the study. Findings are a result of an inductive–deductive interaction between this conceptualization and what you find in the data. The time to prepare for this interaction is in the proposal writing, where you offer a plan for analysis and interpretation.

The analytic framework is embedded in your conceptual framework—that is, in the perspectives, research, and theories from which you developed the rationale and purpose for the study and built your argument. Out of this framework, you generated research questions, and you drew on this framework to identify a generative design. Once again, these tools—your perspective, reviewed research, and theoretical orientations as well as the design elements—contribute to shaping an initial framework to guide data collection, analysis, and interpretation. What happens once you begin data collection will continue to inform this preliminary analytic framework.

The analytic framework Samira uses will be guided by theories and perspectives on which she based her conceptualization. The sensitizing concepts that she identifies will suggest survey or interview questions as well as categories or variables for analysis. If she focuses on retention theories that emphasize both background and assimilation, she will ask students questions about their families, their high school experience, and how they become involved in college life. If she chooses to focus on critical race theory, her questions will be directed toward experiences related to race, laws, and power. Her analyses will document and seek patterns in and among these categories or variables.

Similarly, these concepts influence the design she chooses, which, in turn, shapes the analytic framework. For a descriptive design, she would identify categories of characteristics that she would analyze through surveys, observations, interviews, or artifacts. She would then build representations using numbers, words, terms, phrases, pictures. Should she want to seek relationships between background and graduation, she would propose a correlation study; the analytic framework would specify the variables for which she would measure degree of association. Whatever her design and method, Samira's planning at the proposal stage for how she will analyze and interpret the data will prepare her to conduct a trustworthy study with potentially usable findings.

THE RESEARCH PROPOSAL: BRINGING IT ALL TOGETHER

Thus far, we have worked through the relationship between the conceptual framework and the design and have considered the flow from overall design to research methods, albeit briefly. All this hard intellectual work has involved exciting insights, back-and-forths, frustrations, and, we hope, some clarity for your inquiry project. We now briefly discuss how all these are brought together in a formal research proposal. What you have been doing up to now is thinking, practicing, trying out ideas; now is the time to make your thinking concrete in a written proposal (although we hope you've been drafting preliminary sections all along). What we discuss next is necessarily brief because many excellent texts offer guidance on the details of proposals. Also note that the exact organization of your proposal will depend on the norms in your discipline and the reviewers/readers of your proposal. Although many of you will submit proposals to your faculty committee, others may be submitting proposals to funding agencies or to both. Whatever your audience (discussed further in Chapter 8), there are key aspects of your proposed inquiry project that any reader wants to know. We outline these next. In many disciplines, these are organized as chapters; in others, they may be sections. Also, in some disciplines, the norms are that the proposal include a full review of the literature; in others, a synthesis of key research and theories is required—all, of course, demonstrating that there is a gap that your proposed research will address.

Think of a proposal as an argument that should convince the reader that the study is do-able, potentially significant, and well crafted and that you are competent to conduct it (Marshall & Rossman, 2011). The key aspects of your project that a reader must learn about are, fundamentally, the *what* and the *how*. First, of course, you begin with an *introduction*, which should briefly discuss the following: the larger issue that the research is about, the focus for your specific inquiry, how this study may be potentially significant, and the design and methods (an overview). In Chapter 7, we offer a bit more detail on the importance of the introduction as well as some specific suggestions for making it engaging.

After the introduction, the proposal moves into the *conceptual framework*, the *what*, which provides the reader with the following:

- The *topic*;
- The *statement of the problem*: how this topic relates to larger issues, including background on the issue or problem;
- The *purpose* of the proposed study: what you intend to accomplish;
- The *potential significance* of the study: how the study may contribute to the discourses in your field, to policy, to practice;
- The *review of the literature*: what the currents of thought are that your study links to and is situated within; what key concepts are and how you are defining them; what is known and where gaps are;
- *Research questions*: grand tour and subquestions, hypotheses you intend to test;
- *Analytic framework*: key ideas, concepts, hypotheses that emerge from the conceptual framework and will guide data analysis and interpretation; and
- *Limitations* of the study.

Next, the *design and methods* section, the *how*, provides the following details for the reader:

- The *overall design/approach* and rationale: how this design will be useful and generative, why this design is appropriate;
- *Sampling strategies*: from whom/what, and when, data will be gathered;
- *Data-gathering methods*: how you will generate or access data that will respond to the research questions or test the hypotheses;
- *Data analysis and interpretation procedures*: how you will analyze and interpret the data, based on the analytic framework, to generate responses to the research questions, given your purpose;
- *Trustworthiness*: procedures you will implement to ensure that the study is valid, credible, and robust; and
- *Ethical considerations*: how you will protect human subjects, if you are using them as sources of data.

As you develop a full proposal (or even a mini-proposal), think about how the key ideas or hypotheses developed from the various literatures (the conceptual framework) need to be visible throughout the document. That is, the reader should be able to see clearly how key ideas have led to the research questions; then how these questions inform the choice of design and methods; and finally how the loop is closed through the analytic framework. There should be integrity—wholeness, elegance, and simplicity—in the overall argument presented in the proposal. In our experience, all too often the conceptual framework and research questions are disconnected from the design, methods, and analysis plan. Be sure to link these together for a coherent argument!

AN EXAMPLE OF CONNECTING
THE *WHAT* AND THE *HOW*

To illustrate how the *what* and *how* pieces of the puzzle fit together, we draw on the dissertation of another student we have taught, Ian Martin (2010). Ian had been a director of counseling in a school district before coming to the university to work on his doctorate. He was interested in factors that supported program improvement and used his coursework to explore various literatures on reform and change for improvement. Among the many theories and approaches he learned, he was drawn to program evaluation as a practice that could support organizational learning and improvement. He found research that suggested how evaluation purposes and participatory practices could build capacity for program improvement. From his reading he constructed a theoretical framework. Figure 6.2 depicts a summary of this framework.

Ian then turned to explore whether or how counseling programs used evaluation and decided to focus on state-level school counseling efforts. His review revealed that few states in the United States evaluate their counseling programs. Thus, his argument and purpose:

Argument and Purpose

Given specific purposes and participatory practices, program evaluation can serve to support program improvement. However, few

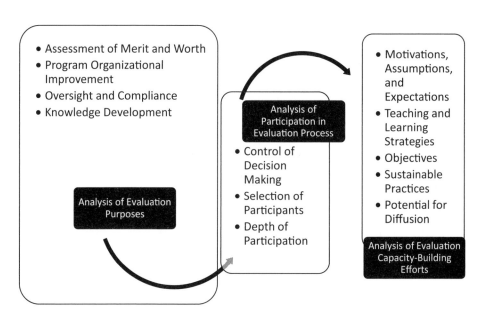

FIGURE 6.2. Ian's theoretical framework. The model is based on Mark, Henry, and Julnes (2000); Cousins and Whitmore (1998); and Preskill and Boyle (2008).

states in the United States are currently evaluating their school counseling programs. Three states with established school counseling programs were identified in the literature as having systemwide evaluation schemas. This study aims to learn from these cases how evaluation may be used in supporting and sustaining state-level school counseling programs.

From the expressed purpose, Ian articulated research questions:

Research Questions

What lessons can be learned from analyzing exemplary cases of state-supported program evaluation?

1. How and why do exemplary cases evaluate their programs?
2. How do exemplary states involve participants in program evaluation?
3. How have exemplary programs built evaluation capacity within their states?

His design (the *how*) choice logically followed his questions and conceptual framework (the *what*); he would conduct descriptive and exploratory case studies. Eventually, Ian decided to compare and contrast similarities and differences across the cases. The following depicts his approach and summarizes his plan for analysis.

Design and Methods

A mixed method cross-case analysis design was selected. The study consisted of three phases:

1. Document review, telephone interviews, and online questionnaires of 389 practicing school counselors.
2. Travel to states for observations, in-depth interviews of key participants, and initial construction of individual case studies.
3. Analysis through lenses of purpose (merit and worth; program improvement; oversight; development); participation (decision

making; selection—who and how; depth); capacity building (expectations and objectives; professional development; resource allocation).

4. Secondary analysis of similarities and differences in purposes, participation, and capacity building between the cases.

We are happy to report that Ian's reading, thinking, and writing during the proposal stage prepared him well for his survey development, fieldwork, and data analysis and interpretation. Surely, he encountered surprises and challenges, but he was able to adjust and modify. For example, one of the states did not work out as a site for research, so his dissertation described and compared only two states as cases. He received his degree in August 2010.

Our goal in this chapter has been to illustrate the connection between your conceptual framework with your emergent research questions and possible designs with appropriate methods. To that end, we discussed purposes and provided a brief overview of various research designs and a short discussion of some research methods. Before turning to the important topic of research use and audiences in Chapter 8, however, we digress a bit in Chapter 7 to offer you some considerations about writing. We see conceptual development as intimately linked with writing; thus, we give this topic some space there. We also address the difficult issue of plagiarism, an all-too-frequent form of academic dishonesty. We then turn, in Chapter 8, to discussions about ways to encourage use of the findings of your inquiry projects.

Learning Activity 6.1. What's the Purpose Here?

To help you critically "read" research statements and questions, we offer sample mini-vignettes and invite you, in your triads, to figure out what the purpose of each study might be. We have found that this helps you become clearer about the purpose of your own inquiry projects and to make sound inferences from what others have written. Following are four examples; we update these regularly, often with examples from a previous class's work.

1. A researcher working at the intersection of psychology and environmental studies is intrigued with the value commitments of individuals who produce little to no trash. He poses the following research question: "What do individuals who are extremely committed to environmental issues do in their everyday lives?" How would you describe the purpose of this study?

2. How would you describe the purpose of an online, survey-based study with the title "An Investigation into the Daily Practices of Human Rights Activists"?

3. How would you classify the purpose of an adolescent psychologist's study titled "An Investigation of the Relationship Between Perfectionism and Anorexia"?

4. What might be the purpose behind this research question: "What percentage of first-year students graduate from college within 5 years?"

Learning Activity 6.2. Scripting My Study

We invite you to work through the following script to help you get clear about their purpose and some aspects of their designs (adapted from Rossman & Rallis, 2012, p. 130). The script is unwieldy as a narrative style, but can help you clarify your focus.

The purpose of my study is to _____ (describe? explore? explain? predict? compare?) the _____ (central idea, concept) for _____ (the unit of analysis: individual person? group? interactions? event?) using a _____ (in-depth interview? RCT? survey?) design and _____ (interviews? questionnaires? Q-sort? archival analysis?) research methods.

Learning Activity 6.3. Will My Study Be Do-able?

Select one or two of your developing research questions. For each question, ask yourself:

- If I want to pursue this question, what information do I need?
- From whom or from where might I gather that information?

- If it involves people, are they likely to be willing?
- How might I gather or obtain it?
- From whom do I need permission?
- Do I need a "sponsor"?
- What about gatekeepers?

FOR FURTHER READING

Cone, J. D., & Foster, S. L. (2006). *Dissertations and theses from start to finish: Psychology and related fields* (2nd ed.). Washington, DC: American Psychological Association.

Creswell, J. W. (2008). *Research design: Qualitative, quantitative, and mixed methods approaches* (3rd ed.). Thousand Oaks, CA: Sage.

Creswell, J. W., & Plano Clark, V. L. (2010). *Designing and conducting mixed methods research* (2nd ed.). Thousand Oaks, CA: Sage.

Hesse-Biber, S. N., & Leavy, P. (Eds.). (2008). *Handbook of emergent methods*. New York: Guilford Press.

Kline, R. B. (2008). *Becoming a behavioral science researcher: A guide to producing research that matters*. New York: Guilford Press.

Mason, J. (2011). *Understanding social research: Thinking creatively about method*. Thousand Oaks, CA: Sage.

Mertens, D. M. (Ed.). (2009). *Research and evaluation in education and psychology* (3rd ed.). Thousand Oaks, CA: Sage.

Patton, M. Q. (2010). *Developmental evaluation: Applying complexity concepts to enhance innovation and use*. New York: Guilford Press.

Roberts, C. M. (2010). *The dissertation journey: A practical and comprehensive guide to planning, writing, and defending your dissertation* (2nd ed.). Thousand Oaks, CA: Sage.

CHAPTER 7

Things to Consider in Writing

Staying in the Right Lane

Critical Questions to Guide Your Reading

- *Why are introductions important? (remembering)*
- *What do I need to know about my audience? (understanding)*
- *What are the principles and practices to avoid plagiarism? (remembering)*
- *How can I use exercises to free up my writing for this inquiry project? (applying)*
- *How will I know that a critical friend has provided useful feedback? (evaluating)*
- *How should I begin my introduction? (creating)*

Dialogue 7. Being Clear to Others

Professor Bettara's students have reviewed each other's draft mini-literature reviews. These papers were challenging for them to write, as each encountered difficulties in getting clear about their arguments and the points they were trying to make. As they gathered into their small group, they vented their frustrations.

REILLY: OK, you guys. It's hard to admit... I need help on how I begin this dumb paper. I'm not sure I've made my big point clear enough. Can we start with me?

SAMIRA: Sure, but maybe we should begin by each person saying what they'd most like to get from this feedback. Would that work? I think Reilly wants to focus on his introduction, right?

MARTINA: I think so . . . I've got other problems, like with the problem statement. It's really hard, with English being my fourth language, to be so direct and explicit, like I think Bettara wants. Where I come from, things are left kind of unstated.

KEVIN: Yeah, well, I'm having trouble figuring out the balance between being more personal and being more "academic." Bettara always wants us to open up our writing, but now I'm really confused. And this lit review isn't like those early papers we did. Remember when we wrote a letter to a friend? That was way easier for me.

RAUL: I guess I'm into all those periods and quotation marks and commas and spaces. This "APA" is killing me!

SAMIRA: What concerns me most is making it interesting. I don't want to just list my sources, or a boring annotated bibliography. Bettara warned us not to do that.

RAUL: Same here. How do we integrate, or "synthesize"—using Bettara's words—into a coherent whole?

KEVIN: Before I worry about whether my paper is interesting, I worry about all this citation and plagiarism stuff. I've heard stories about students getting kicked out for not following the rules about giving credit for other people's words. Easy to say, but how do I do it? I mean, I've read all this stuff so, of course, I'm going to use others' words. I'm confused.

REILLY: Hey, remember me? Can we just start with how I make my introduction clear?

This dialogue represents one of the major concerns looming over any student new to academia (and many veterans as well): how to hook their readers and write papers that both are interesting and meet the requirements of their discipline. This short chapter highlights some considerations in writing. As we noted earlier, thinking, reflecting, and writing are deeply intertwined. We have our students write and write and then write some more as a strategy for helping them get clear about their ideas. There are, however, some key areas where focused instruction and practice can help out. In this chapter, we discuss writing introductions, the tricky (and painful) issue of plagiarism, and standard citation systems.

WRITING INTRODUCTIONS

Why do we begin at the beginning, with writing introductions? Quite simply, if you don't engage your readers right away, you lose them. If readers are obligated to read your work (e.g., your professor), this may not be as important as when you write a policy brief, a scholarly journal article, a grant proposal, or even a short piece for a newspaper. Engaging your readers *right away* means that these people may actually continue on to read your entire piece. If readers are not engaged, the introduction may be all that they read, and your work will fail to make any impression on policy, your discipline, a funding source, the public. Given our commitment to use, this seems like a waste of your—and your readers'—time. We next offer some pointers on writing strong, inviting introductions.

> Introductions matter because they capture the reader's attention.

Questions to Address

Think about really fascinating novels that you have read. What did the authors do? Most likely, they grabbed you quickly into an exciting or problematic situation or set of interactions. The result? You want to know more, so you read on. Just as with novels, your paper needs to invite readers into your thinking, telling them what you are focusing on (the larger issue or topic) and then what is problematic or complicated about this. To do this, set up an unproblematic but perhaps dramatic set of circumstances, one that establishes common ground with the readers, and then *complicate* or *disrupt* it. Then go on to describe how your inquiry project may help with *a solution* to the problem and why this matters. We elaborate on these elements shortly; for now, it may be useful to think about how your introduction should respond to the following questions:

- What are you focusing on? [larger issue/topic]
- What is the problematic situation? [complication, disruption]
- How might your research contribute or help? [response]
- Why does this matter? [consequence, potential significance]

Common Elements

The typical elements of an introduction are a contextualizing background, a statement of the problem, and your response to the problem. The *contextualizing background*, as just noted, establishes common ground with the reader, focuses on the larger issue, and is typically unproblematic. An example from Samira might read:

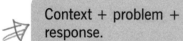

Context + problem + response.

> Minority populations are projected to become the majority in the United States by 2030.

This is unproblematic in the sense that the readers are likely to agree (however, Samira will have to support this assertion with data—evidence—in the body of her paper).

Readers are then likely to ask themselves, "What is problematic about this?" The *statement of the problem* disrupts the readers' sense of a somewhat stable context—it problematizes that context, drawing out a more specific focus for the paper. Use words such as *however, but, in spite of,* and *nevertheless* to signal to the readers that all is not well. Samira might write:

> However, despite their growing numbers, minority students are graduating from college at lower and lower rates.

Note her use of *however* and *despite* to signal a complication that the readers (she hopes) should pay attention to.

Samira will then go on to state,

Words or phrases such as *however, but, in spite of*, and *nevertheless* signal complications.

While we can document the increasing numbers of minority students who drop out, we do not know why. If we do not address this issue, the potential for this population to contribute to the economy and social well-being will be lost.

In this statement, Samira is setting up a *condition of incomplete knowledge* or understanding and establishing the *consequences* of that condition. She will then provide her response by indicating how her research will help address the consequences—by filling the gap in knowledge or by helping to solve the problem. Samira's introduction might then look like this:

Minority populations are projected to become the majority in the United States by 2030. However, despite their growing numbers, minority students are graduating from college at lower and lower rates. While we can document the increasing numbers of minority students who drop out, we do not know why. If we do not address this issue, the potential for this population to contribute to the economy and social well-being will be lost. To help address this situation, my research will analyze the student pathways through college at two small liberal arts colleges: one that is successful and one that is not. Such comparisons will deepen our understanding of what types of support help minority students to persevere.

Another example may help, this one about a study of Fair Trade coffee growers and potential consequences to those living in poverty. The first statement establishes common ground and contextualizes the topic for the reader:

Fair Trade certification links ethically minded consumers to cooperatively organized small farmers.

This assertion then should be complicated:

However, participation in cooperatives, rather than large-scale plantations, demands increased labor.

What are the likely consequences of this problematic situation?

Households may, therefore, not be able to use the full resources of the cooperative, which may lead to continued cycles of poverty.

How will this potential consequence be addressed, and how might this study contribute?

> This research will study a successful small farmers' cooperative, thereby contributing to our understanding of the factors that support such success.

With these examples in mind, we now offer some tips on how *not* to begin an introduction.

How *Not* to Start

We have observed two common ways to begin that don't work well. One is beginning with a *dictionary definition*:

> Power Distance is defined by . . . as . . .

Another is by starting with grandiose claims that end up inviting the reader to disagree with you and not be interested in reading further:

> The most famous psychologists have struggled with the topic of group morality.

Good Ways to Start

There are several approaches to writing an effective introduction. One is to present *a striking fact* about your topic, as Samira did in the example given earlier:

> Shellfish remains are found in over 83% of the landmass of the islands of southern New England.

> Celebrity gossip blogs increased over 3,000% between 2001 and 2008.

 Another is to begin with *an engaging quotation*:

> "Never send to know for whom the bell tolls; it tolls for thee." (John Donne, Meditation 17)

"Be not conformed to this world: but be ye transformed by the renewing of your mind." (Romans 12:2)

Note, however, that the quote must be *directly* related to your topic. Don't use a quote just because you like it! Yet another effective way to begin is with *an appropriate anecdote*:

Kathy and Jennifer entered the courtroom filled with misgivings. Iris, their 2-year-old daughter, might be taken away from them by the court.

> **Remember: You can deal with a reader who disagrees with you. You cannot deal with a reader who doesn't care or doesn't understand.**

More Tips and Considerations

Audience, audience, audience. Another way to say this is, reader, reader, reader. To engage your readers effectively, you need to know something about them, or you need to imagine what their values and interests are. If you are writing for a professor, learn as much as you can about his or her expectations for the paper. If you are writing for a scholarly journal, read previous issues to see the preferred tone, style, and subject matter. If you are writing a grant proposal, find out the funder's values and interests. Your primary task in an introduction is to convince the readers that what you are writing about is important and fascinating!

We turn now to a much more difficult topic: plagiarism. Put more positively, this issue comes under the broad category of "academic honesty." Recall the discussion in Chapter 4 about how readers—the audience for your work—must trust in the soundness and rigor of your work. Readers must also trust that it is *your* work. This is the foundation on which scholarship is built. The next section discusses some of the issues associated with plagiarism and offers some examples.

THE NASTY PROBLEM OF PLAGIARISM[5]

As a university student, either undergraduate or graduate, you will write term papers, comprehensive examinations, theses, and/or dissertations. One way or another, these written pieces will draw on the work of many other

---

[5] This section draws from Rossman and Evans (2002), with permission from the authors.

authors. Being able to draw on other authors' work is a skill that you must master in order to navigate your way through the university effectively. In Western contexts, the rules governing how and when you use the ideas and words of others are taken very seriously. If you don't learn these rules—and if you violate them, either wittingly or unwittingly—there can be serious consequences. You can, for example, be removed from the university, or a finding of plagiarism can become part of your permanent academic record.

A Cultural Critique

Different cultures have varying assumptions about how knowledge is created and legitimated, and varying norms about how other authors' words and ideas should appropriately be used. Western cultures are highly individualistic and typically place a good deal of emphasis on *intellectual property*, that is, the individual's ownership of ideas and written words. Thus, written words and ideas are viewed as belonging to the individual who wrote them. For students from other cultures, this is a difficult set of assumptions to grasp. Majority world students often come from cultures where one's experiences, thoughts, and ideas are intermingled with those of others, so the notion of "owning" ideas is anathema. However, if you are studying in a Western university, you must master these principles. In Western contexts, one author's words can *never* be used by another author without explicitly acknowledging the source (through the citation systems discussed next).

> Don't plagiarize . . . ever. When in doubt, ask.

Using the Work of Other Authors

There are three ways to draw upon the writings of other authors: summarizing, paraphrasing, or quoting directly. Each way demands that you acknowledge that the ideas or words are not your own. The fundamental principle guiding the use of others' work has two components: (1) identifying what is not your own work (i.e., referring to the author of the ideas or words) and (2) providing the source from which those ideas or words came.

When you *summarize* a major point, main argument, position, or perspective of an author, you should reference that author and her work as a whole, without providing specific page numbers. An example:

> In his generative work *Pedagogy of the Oppressed*, Freire (1970) develops a theory that explains the psychology of oppression and its effects on both the oppressed and the oppressor.

If you summarize ideas that are taken for granted and well known in your field, you may not need to cite specific authors, but you should check with others (e.g., professors or advisors) about that. When, however, you make claims about specific facts (population figures, demographic data), you *must* provide a reference to a specific source. Why? So that your readers can check the source and data or go to those sources for their own learning.

Quite often, as you write, you will *paraphrase* the words or elements of an argument of other authors. When you paraphrase, you describe the other author's ideas but in your own words. In so doing, you are distilling and interpreting what that author has written. When paraphrasing, you should be careful that you are accurately representing what the author wrote while placing emphasis on those elements of his work that you want to highlight. When you paraphrase another author's ideas or words, you must provide a reference to the work, with page numbers for accuracy. An example:

> From Freire's perspective, when poor people resort to violence, they are not the aggressors. For him, violent actions have their roots in the oppressive structures which cause extreme poverty (1970, p. 41).

In this example, note the use of the phrases "From Friere's perspective" and "For him." These rhetorical devices signal that you are paraphrasing. Also note the specific page reference. This facilitates the reader turning to the source, locating that page, and reading Freire's words herself.

Finally, as you write, you will *quote directly* from other authors because their particular language is evocative and expressive, and it captures the points eloquently. When doing so, keep these direct quotations short. Remember that the purpose of writing a paper is to demonstrate your thinking and analysis of the key ideas that frame your topic. The discussion in Chapter 5 about conceptualizing and writing a literature review is relevant here: Do not provide long, direct quote after long, direct quote. The reader wants to see how you understand these ideas. Thus, strive for balance between your own analysis and words and those of others.

> Those who try to free others by telling them that they are oppressed or exhorting them with slogans are, in Freire's eyes, trying to "liberate the oppressed with the instruments of domestication" (1970, p. 29).

Giving credit where credit is due—to the ideas, arguments, words of others—is enacted through specific rules, or citation systems. Different disciplines rely on different citation systems; in the next section, we provide a short discussion of one system—that of the American Psychological Association—as an example. Citation systems are the "nuts and bolts" of crediting the work of others.

USING PROPER CITATION FORMAT

Learning the citation system that your discipline or department customarily uses is important. Although these rules seem at times arbitrary, you must master them early on. We moan over dissertation proposals in which the student still is getting citation formatting wrong! Remember to think about your reader: Will it impress a professor that, after several years of graduate study, you have not yet mastered these simple, albeit strange, rules? Of course not. So master whichever style your discipline uses.

> Master your discipline's citation system— practice it early and often until it is a routine part of your writing.

Because we work in the social sciences, we use the American Psychological Association's style rules, commonly referred to as APA. The association publishes various manuals and guidelines for those who need to learn and use the APA style of citations. Their materials also include excellent discussions of integrity in writing, hints for crisp and succinct writing styles, and strategies for avoiding plagiarism, as well as considerations of gender-neutral language and grammar. We recommend that you go to *www.apastyle.org* for the most recent resources on writing and on citation rules. There is also software that you can use with word-processing programs that will automatically format citations in the text and in the reference list properly, for example, EndNote™ (*www.endnote.com*), a commercially available system that you can install on your computer, and RefWorks™ (*www.refworks.com*), a Web-based, centrally managed system typically supported by university libraries.

We will not go through even the most used citation formats here; there are many sources available to help you learn those. Our advice is to learn the citation system most commonly used in your discipline or field and master the specifics. Although this will seem tedious and perhaps pointless, mastering the system early in your academic career will save you much time later.

Audience, introductions, plagiarism, proper citation—these considerations will help you develop an argument that is elegant, persuasive, and compelling. Having worked through these, we turn next in Chapter 8 to thinking about use. We have argued throughout this book that grounding your inquiry projects in real-world concerns, issues, puzzles, or curiosities is crucial for ensuring that your work will not sit unread on a library shelf, in a database repository, or on a coffee table. We turn to these now.

Learning Activities 7.1. Freeing Up Your Writing

We often find that students are "tight" with their writing. Thus, in addition to writing the position papers on topics that fascinate you (see Chapter 5), we encourage you to try out several strategies.

- *Talk to a critical friend.* Talking through your ideas can sometimes help clarify them. Be sure that your conversational partner will ask you "critical" questions—questions that ask you to create more clear, elaborate connections in your logic and examine your assumptions. Ask that person to take notes so you have a record of what you said.

- *Talk into a digital tape recorder.* Just as talking with a critical friend can help, so can talking into a tape recorder. This gives you a more complete record than notes taken by your critical friend. You can then listen to the tape and transcribe it.

- *Talk to your grandmother.* This is a reality check. If you can make your ideas clear to someone who cares and is intelligent but not immersed in the jargon of your discipline, you are well on your way to making your ideas clear to readers—your audience.

- *Create a collage of your ideas.* With a variety of art materials (e.g., scraps of paper, markers, twine, glitter), create a nonverbal depiction of your emerging ideas. What do the scraps, for example, represent? How do they connect? What do you want to foreground and background? We have found that using nonverbal representations can bring new insights.

Learning Activity 7.2. Analyzing Writing

- *Analyze the argument in a journal article in your field.* Identify an important article in your field from a respected journal. Read first for content: What are the main points? What "sticks" after you are finished reading? Then reread for the argument: What are the central assertions? What evidence is put forward to support those claims? How does the evidence connect with the assertions (the warrants)? Where is the author in the text? And how does the author "hedge" her points? Noting these subtle but powerful rhetorical devices will help you learn to incorporate them into your own writing.

- *Analyze the use of metaphor in a journal article in your field.* Identify an article. As in the previous activity, first read for content. Then reread, this time paying particular attention to the metaphors the author uses. Metaphors often escape our direct attention but have a powerful effect on how we understand the author's points and perspective. Metaphors come up in verbs (*"building* an argument"), in adjectives (*"warm* spots and *cool* spots"), in nouns ("the *foundation* of this field").

- *Rewrite a paper you wrote previously.* Take a paper that you wrote for a previous class. It's best to use one that you have some "distance" from. Conduct a critical analysis: How does the organization of the paper flow? What key assertions did you make? How did you support them? Were the transitions from one section to another clear? Did they lead the reader on logically? In recommending this activity, we caution students against being too critical of their own work. It is quite easy to think, "Did *I* write this? It's awful!" Be gentle on yourself—you are learning the skills of self-editing, which will stand you in good stead with any writing project.

FOR FURTHER READING

➡ Beard, R., Myhill, D., Riley, J., & Nystrand, M. (Eds.). (2009). *The Sage handbook of writing development*. London: Sage.

➡ Booth, W. C., Colomb, G. G., & Williams, J. M. (2008). *The craft of research* (3rd ed.). Chicago: University of Chicago Press.

➡ Corbett, E. P. J., Finkle, S. L., & Myers, N. (2008). *The little English handbook: Choices and conventions* (8th ed.). New York: Pearson Longman.

➡ Harris, R. A. (2011). *Using sources effectively: Strengthening your writing and avoiding plagiarism* (3rd ed.). Glendale, CA: Pyrczak.

➡ Nash, R. L. (2004). *Liberating scholarly writing: The power of personal narrative*. New York: Teachers College Press.

➡ Plotnik, A. (2007). *Spunk and bite: A writer's guide to bold, contemporary style*. New York: Random House.

➡ Richardson, L. (1990). *Writing strategies: Reaching diverse audiences*. Thousand Oaks, CA: Sage.

➡ Strunk, W., Jr., & White, E. B. (2010). *The elements of style* (4th ed.). New York: Harlow Pearson.

➡ Truss, L. (2003). *Eats, shoots and leaves: The zero tolerance approach to punctuation*. New York: Gotham Books.

➡ Ven Leunen, M.-C. (1992). *A handbook for scholars: A complete guide to the mechanics of scholarly writing* (rev. ed.). New York: Oxford University Press.

➡ Zinsser, W. (2006). *On writing well: The classic guide to writing nonfiction* (7th ed., rev. & updated). New York: HarperCollins.

CHAPTER 8

Knowledge Use
Arriving at Your Destination

⊛ *Critical Questions to Guide Your Reading*

➥ *What ways can knowledge be used? (remembering)*

➥ *Why is use important? (understanding)*

➥ *What are potential audiences for my inquiry project? (applying)*

➥ *How do I communicate with different audiences? (applying)*

➥ *What does passion have to do with my project and use? (understanding)*

➥ *How might I ensure use of my project? (creating)*

Dialogue 8. How Can the Results of Our Inquiry Be Used for Improvement?

The semester is ending, and the five students we have followed throughout are meeting together before the final inquiry class, when Professor Bettara will return their mini-project proposals.

MARTINA: I'm glad we are getting our proposals back today. I really want to see what Bettara thinks of my ideas.

KEVIN: Well, not me. I'm not sure I want to see the feedback. I'm just glad it's over.

SAMIRA: You two . . . talking about feedback. Sure, I want to know what the professor thinks, but I'm going to do something like what I proposed whatever Bettara says. I really want low-income minority students to persist in college so I need to learn what influences them. It's a social justice issue. If we know what empowers students, then we can make changes to help them.

REILLY: It's not that easy. You're assuming a direct link between any changes you make and students' attitudes and behavior.

MARTINA: But we all want our findings to be used . . . and used to improve, as Bettara says, the "human condition." The children in the villages whose parents have died from AIDS need help. I want to learn something that will contribute to their getting that help.

SAMIRA: Isn't that Reilly's point? There may not be a direct connection between your findings and positive changes in these kids' lives. Maybe all you can do is draw attention to the situation and their needs.

RAUL: Yeah. Any finding, that is, information, becomes knowledge only when someone uses it. So, I wonder, who will use my findings? And how? Seriously, most research just sits on shelves. For example, who ever reads dissertations? Besides, you realize, it's possible that findings could even be used in negative ways.

MARTINA: I never thought of that, but it is so true. Given the political situation surrounding AIDS and the villages, one side could interpret my findings to suit their position, and that could be very different from what I intended.

KEVIN: I suppose it matters how we report our findings. And you are right that nobody will read my dissertation . . . and I'm not sure I'll want anyone to! Of course, I don't have to worry about any of my colleagues reading whatever I write. I'll certainly have to find other ways to communicate whatever I learn about.

RAUL: You know, I'm thinking how I might create a video game based on my findings.

REILLY: A game sure would reach a broader audience than a boring old report. Just think: If research findings were disseminated through more popular media, it would level out the playing field, pun intended. Seriously, only a privileged sector has access to research findings now.

SAMIRA: Good ideas, but we'd better do the research and write our dissertations first!

The group continues to talk, considering who might be interested in what they discover and how they might communicate their learning.

So here you are; you've arrived at what appears to be the end of your journey. You've designed and implemented a study; you've collected, analyzed, and interpreted data. You have informed your question and have learned something—in terms of both your question and the research process. But have you produced knowledge yet? Doesn't the information you have in your findings need to be used before it becomes knowledge? How can what you learned contribute, in some way, to improving the human condition? Perhaps you are not quite finished with your journey because you still have several questions: Who might use your research findings? How do people use the results of research? What does use look like? As well, you might be wondering how to reach those who might be interested, how to best communicate your findings.

Throughout the book, we have considered what knowledge is and how knowledge is generated. Now this final dialogue among the student learners strikes at the importance of use: To become knowledge, information must be used, and its use should in some way contribute to improving the human condition. Using information, however, is more complicated than may appear at first glance. What does it mean to use information? Who uses information? How do they use it? Does everyone use knowledge in the same way? How can the way the information is communicated promote or hinder use? Because you have spent a semester becoming an inquiry-minded graduate student, you already expect that the answers to these questions are not simple. Just as there are multiple ways of knowing, there are multiple ways to communicate information and use knowledge. This chapter raises questions of use, audience, communication of findings, and contribution to a larger social good. We explore different forms use may take, as well as the influences on how your findings may be used. These influences include your original purposes of the inquiry; the nature of your discoveries; potential audiences; how you communicate what you learned; and, of course, your passion for findings.

USING WHAT YOU HAVE LEARNED

We have presented inquiry as a learning process, and our focus has been on *systematic inquiry*, a patterned and deliberative process involving decisions about the questions, evidence, data collection, making meaning of the data, and audiences. Decisions are also made about documenting and reporting the rationale and process so relevant communities may judge the adequacy of the study and the trustworthiness of the findings. Through systematic inquiry, a researcher moves—not always directly—from assertions to arguments to literature reviews to conceptualizations to designing and conducting a study that *may* produce knowledge.

We emphasize the *"may* produce" over *"does* produce" knowledge because we all realize that a lot of research merely sits on shelves, unread and unused. Naturally, we would like to think that most people conduct studies with the aim of improving programs and practices, but a common complaint heard among practitioners is that research findings do not really inform practice. A gap between production and use is more common than a direct link. In practice, the perceived gap may be due to a misunderstanding of how we use information.

Instrumental Use

Traditionally, the most commonly expressed reason for conducting research is intended instrumental use—concrete findings will be applied to specific problems to provide solutions or recommendations. The assumption is that findings will be linked directly to actions. Several models fit this linear use:

1. A problem is recognized or identified, but sufficient information is lacking to enact a solution. Research findings inform the problem, and a solution is discovered. Knowledge is produced when the information is used to solve the problem.

   A problem identified → research conducted → findings generated → solution discovered and applied → problem solved

2. A particular goal is sought, but many potential pathways to the goal exist. Research is conducted to find and then test the alternatives so that the best approach can be used to reach the goal. In this model, the goal drives the research and the use of the findings.

> **Instrumental use: Intended use by intended users.**

Goal → identify alternative approaches → test alternatives → generate results → select and apply → goal attained

3. A body of information exists but its application to a problem is unclear. Research is conducted to explore how the information can be applied to the problem. Often, this development of existing information can provide solutions to other problems.

Information → research and development → application to problem

Each of these models represents *intended use by intended users*,[6] and each assumes that the connection between problems and solutions is linear, direct, measurable, and rational. For example, Kevin wants to know exactly what a middle school principal can do to support the academic learning of boys. His research is designed to provide specific answers that he can use; thus, he intends to use his findings instrumentally.

Enlightenment Use

In reality, however, enlightenment use is more common. We argue that in practice very few research findings are used as directly and rationally as instrumental use implies. More often, people use information less consciously, with the link between any research findings and human action less observable or attributable. Instead, people accumulate information that ultimately contributes to a gradual reorientation, a deeper understanding or insight. The information accumulates slowly so that identifying which specific information forms the basis of any decision or action is impossible. Usually, one piece of information contributes to several decisions, and any decision is reached through multiple sources of information. Information contributes to general knowledge, enhances understanding, offers heuristic insight. Put simply, information serves to enlighten people's thinking and actions.

---

[6]While Michael Q. Patton uses this phrase in his book *Utilization-Focused Evaluation* (2008), our meaning is slightly different.

Accumulated knowledge from research findings improves practice because it builds practitioners' insights into the principles behind their pro-

cedures. Most practitioners recognize that what they do is the result of information they have collected over the years. In schooling, for example, balanced reading instruction (both phonics and whole language approaches) is a practice that has been enlightened by research knowledge. Many teachers held the philosophy and practiced the approach long before they heard the term. As they read the emerging literature on balanced reading, they acquired insights into the principles behind their practices and thus enhanced their teaching. Similarly, when making diagnoses, physicians draw on the vast body of information that they have acquired over the years.

> Enlightenment use: Information accumulates.

A classic example of how information accumulates to change the way people think about an issue comes from the field of mental health. Rein (1970) describes how a series of controversial and threatening reports of treatment of patients in a mental hospital were not used by the organization itself to improve services; the reports were, however, read by others in the mental health field. As more people read and identified with the reported treatment, a gradual change occurred in the operation of mental hospitals. Similarly, Samira hopes that people who read her stories of the challenges facing college students of color begin to realize the complexity of the experience. She does not expect her stories to provide answers or solutions, but she does believe that, if enough of those readers who come to understand the situation more fully hold positions in institutions of higher education, changes might be made in services and supports for students of color.

SYMBOLIC AND POLITICAL USE

Other uses, while frequent and authentic, are less explicit; these are symbolic and political uses. When findings provide new images to express or represent a situation or phenomenon or to crys-

> Symbolic use: Evokes new and shared images.

tallize shared beliefs or values, the research serves symbolic purposes. Research findings become political when used to shape public perceptions, legislative actions, policy statements, and program design through influence, coercion, leverage, or negotiation.

The information from research can encourage users to reconfigure old patterns and to see familiar pictures in new lights. Findings can offer explanations, "making complex, ambiguous experiences and beliefs comprehensible and communicable to others" (Rossman & Rallis, 2012, p. 20). Explanation and understanding are important human needs (Maslowe, 1970); we tend to look for patterns and create narratives that make sense of the world and its phenomena. Research interpretations can address this need by offering definitions and images of values, myths, and rituals that, once accepted among a social or professional group, serve as a common understanding—a glue—that holds the group together. The shared understandings help explain and make acceptable events or actions within that group. Reporting these findings may also serve to surface deeply disturbing actions that a culture publicly masks. For example, Tracey Kidder's *Old Friends* (1993) raised public awareness of the lonely and isolated lives of the elderly in nursing homes in America. His rich descriptions of one nursing home evoked images that are symbolic of aging in America. Martina may write a book or produce a film that pictures the child heads of household in the African villages where AIDS deaths have taken a toll on families; her images may serve a powerful symbolic purpose by portraying and conveying the realities of these children's lives.

Serving more political purposes, research interpretations may legitimize existing logic, myths, beliefs, or preferences, that is, to support actions already taken or decisions already made. We have all seen examples where the conduct and completion of a study, in and of itself, foster public acceptance of a product, situation, or phenomenon. For example, much of the research done on medical or educational policies serves to advocate for the use of procedures chosen to implement the policies. Most federal programs require evaluations (which are seldom read) to demonstrate accountability. We have heard school personnel use ambiguous findings from evaluations to applaud mediocre programs, reasoning that, because an evaluation was completed every year, the program must be legitimate and it must be good, whatever the actual results. In another area, studies conducted and disseminated by pharmaceutical companies on drugs they manufacture offer notorious examples of research being conducted primarily to influence use of the products. In such cases, the research becomes ritual or ceremony where the process or reporting is more important than the results; the act of *researching* signals that something is being done or the existence of a report serves as proxy for value.

When studying a collective bargaining process, we witnessed a union executive pound heavily on a lengthy tome prepared by the union's research staff that detailed deplorable working conditions in the organization. When we interviewed the executive, we learned that he had not read any of the report but declared, "We have research to support our position." The company executive then referred to an economic report prepared by his research staff that refuted the union findings (we wondered how much of the report *he* had read). The interaction between the opposing executives can be seen as a ritual using research as the sacrament on which each side legitimates itself. These various examples illustrate how important the symbolic and political uses of the conduct and findings of research can be to organizations and individuals. As researchers, we have learned to value such uses, and at the same time we caution against unethical misuse.

Emancipatory Use

Any research also has the potential to be *emancipatory*, when the process of inquiry, action, and reflection—and the knowledge it generates—creates opportunities for action that alters some aspect of society for the better. From this perspective, research is a form of social action; practicing research becomes a source of empowerment for participants in their daily life, and results may transform larger social structures, practices, and relationships. Emancipatory use grows out of Paolo Freire's (1970) *web of praxis*: the belief that the reflection and action implicit in knowledge generation can change—and liberate—practice. As with his research in the 1960s and 1970s on Chilean literacy that involved members of oppressed communities identifying issues of vital importance to them, most research that emancipates or empowers involves those who would be studied; they are participants in the true meaning of the word. Participants raise their own questions and study their own settings; they are not generating knowledge simply to inform or enlighten an academic community. Instead, they collaboratively produce knowledge to improve their work and their lives. Any external researcher present may serve as a facilitator. Participatory action research and feminist studies are usually undertaken for emancipatory uses.

Whatever your expectations for how your learning might be used, be prepared for many possibilities—few being what you had in mind. You may wonder how you can facilitate positive uses. Our response is to think about potential audiences and how you might reach them.

WHO CARES?: POTENTIAL AUDIENCES

Recall your original purposes and ask yourself: What did I learn, and who might be interested? What is the nature of my discoveries, and whom do I want to reach? How would I want people to use them? Let's look at some of the audiences you might consider.

Academia and Scholars

Since you are most likely a student in an institution of higher education, your most obvious audience is your professors; they stipulate their expectations for how you conduct your study and report your findings. As scholars themselves, they are likely to use your research to inform their own (attributing the work to you, we hope). They may suggest that you publish your work in a scholarly journal; thus, you approach another audience, your community of discourse. Raul's study on the relationship between learning and funding sources in nonprofit organizations informs his professor's work on organizational change, so they co-author an article that they submit to *Administrative Science Quarterly*.

Policymakers

Many research studies are designed with an aim to inform policymakers—researchers hope that legislators or agency leaders will seek out research findings that can inform their decision making. In reality, legislators employ staff to do just that, but what research they find depends on their ability to locate and review relevant material. If you want to influence policy, you have to reach the ears of policymakers, who are often driven by constituency preferences and power dynamics. Although policy rhetoric calls for instrumental use, enlightenment or political/symbolic use is more common.

We have found that evaluation as applied research can reach decision makers if the findings are timely and accessible. A colleague who worked for one state's office of legislative oversight often regaled us with instances where the results of her office's research changed the direction of a particular piece of legislation, but she admitted that deadlines were tight and reports needed to be clear, concise, and to the point—that is, readable and succinct. Recently, we have evaluated collaboration across agencies serving institutionalized youth. Because interagency collaboration was a priority of the department of mental health's executive director, she read the evaluation report closely and actively advocated for using the findings. Several of Bettara's students hope eventually to influence policymakers with the results of their research. For example, Samira hopes to enlighten institutional policy that can support retention of students of color in her state's colleges and universities. Martina hopes her portraits of child-headed families will change the policies related to resource distribution in the villages.

Practitioners

Those who contribute to getting the work done, the practitioners, form a large and varied group. Included among practitioners are midlevel bureaucrats who translate policy into procedure; leaders who are charged with choosing and shaping policies and procedures into programs that benefit their organizations, personnel, and clients; and on-site workers who implement the programs. Practitioners are managers, agency staff, principals and superintendents, social workers, therapists, teachers, nurses, doctors, and nurse practitioners—the list goes on and on. Practitioners use research results when it informs their ordinary knowledge (Lindblom & Cohen, 1979), that is, when it makes sense to them and fits their daily practices. The author who reviewed our book *Leading Dynamic Schools: How to Create and Implement Ethical Policies* (Rallis et al., 2008) reveals a common attitude of practitioners toward research—and his reaction to discovering practically useful material:

> I selected this book with the same motivation I felt as a child when I'd eat a vegetable dish—not because it tasted good, but because it was good for me and would make me stronger. I was in for a surprise because what I found in this small volume was an engaging text that will have a lasting influence on how I view policy and the process I'll go through with others in formulating and implementing policies in our school. (Warnock, 2008)

We suspect that his attitude changed as he read because we wrote the book directly for practicing principals. The point is that recognizing your audiences allows you to tailor your delivery of research findings and interpretations to facilitate use. Given potential audiences and uses, how do you communicate what you have learned?

COMMUNICATING FOR USE

Chances are that when you began this journey of inquiry, you were not thinking about how you would communicate your findings. You probably assumed
that a formal report would be required, and you would leave it at that. We
argue that the complex social issues and programs that are the focus of social
science research demand appropriate and relevant forms of representation
to convey the usually sophisticated and subtle insights revealed through the
research. We suggest that the many ways of communicating research can be
grouped into three modes or forms of representation: textual–narrative (both
traditional and alternative), visual–expressive, and dialogical.

Textual–Narrative Representations

Textual–narrative representations are useful to communicate interpretations and findings both internally to participants or funders and to interested external audiences you may want to reach. These representations can
take the form of either the more traditional report or the more postmodern/
feminist portrayals as they express propositional, conceptual knowledge, or
practical knowledge. Propositional ways of knowing are usually expressed
as formal reports, policy briefs, analytic memos and essays, and executive
summaries. Reports in whatever form are most useful when they convey
rich descriptions that are readily interpretable and applicable. Alternative
formats for textual–narrative representations portray images and patterns
through verbal metaphor and include stories, portraits, poetry, scripts, day-
in-the-life glimpses, and vignettes. Posts on blogs and Facebook are surfacing as new and effective ways to communicate what you have learned from
your research. These formats are often more evocative, lifting the reader out
of his daily routine and offering a fresh perspective. Moreover, alternative
formats can explicitly address the question of voice; that is, whose experiences, attitudes, skill acquisition, and perception are represented? Participants may speak directly rather than through the researcher's more neutral
or distant voice. A postmodern or critical narrative seeks not to privilege a
dominant voice or interpretation.

   Whichever format you may chose, written text needs structure to be
readable, and various organizers can be used to provide that structure
(recall the discussion on writing in Chapter 7). Analyses and interpretations
may be presented thematically, chronologically, by variable or procedure;

as cases, models, critical events, or episodes; as life histories; by relevant theoretical constructs to name a few. We have seen dissertations written as novelettes and as instructional manuals. Often research findings are best conveyed through secondary analyses that allow alternative interpretations guided by a specific purpose or perspective. For example, to reach school practitioners, Rallis and Goldring wrote *Principals of Dynamic Schools* (2000) based on Rallis's qualitative case studies and on Goldring's quantitative analyses of the massive *High School and Beyond* data set.

In *A Thrice Told Tale*, Wolf (1992) illustrates the multiple formats that textual–narrative representation may take. An anthropologist who studied village life in Taiwan, Wolf presents three written expressions of the same set of incidents related to a village woman: a fictional account, the research field notes, and an analytic essay. With different emphasis and detail, each account communicates a different perspective on the villagers and life in the village.

Visual–Expressive Representations

Visual–expressive representations present knowledge to both internal and external audiences through nonverbal images, media, artifacts, or performances. These include graphic and plastic art forms such as drawing and painting; song; theater arts; films and video; demonstrations and exhibitions. Multimedia and interactive presentations are possible given current technologies. For example, PhotoVoice or digital storytelling interactively involve participants in data collection, analysis, interpretation, and, finally, presentation. Samira may choose one of these methods to involve college students of color in identifying supports and barriers to their persistence in the institution. Raul may create a video game based on his research findings; this representation could communicate his insights into organizational change subtly but more powerfully than a formal report. The nonverbal descriptions and interpretations that emerge in these representations reveal patterns and images and actions that are often deeply evocative of the "lived" context and can crystallize shared understandings among and across audiences.

Dialogical Representations

Dialogical representations draw on the two other modes and are most useful to convey interpretations or emerging insights to internal audiences such as participants or practitioners of the phenomenon studied. Dialogical conversations rely on words—spoken or written—and on nonverbal expressions. Using this mode, the researcher captures and expresses tacit knowledge embedded in the setting and among the people studied; the researcher recognizes that he may know more than he can say (Polanyi, 1966). Dialogical expressions usually rely on either textual–narrative or visual–expressive representations to trigger the dialogue but quickly embrace conversations, negotiations, and exchanges that yield new understandings and, ideally, altered procedures or actions. As an example, we cite our PowerPoint presentations on collaboration in institutional settings to the leadership team of a department of mental health. The PowerPoint presentations were brief, intended to summarize findings that would spark reaction and dialogue. In fact, each slide prompted conversations that informed decisions and eventually led to program modifications. In another example, a study of bullying among middle school students used PhotoVoice, allowing students opportunities to collect data, define terms, share interpretations; the research activity became, in practice, an intervention. Similarly, Raul's video game could serve as a trigger for dialogical interchange among the organization leaders who play together. In summary, dialogical representation facilitates movement beyond the obvious, the expected, the scripted.

With so many ways to communicate what you have learned, you may wonder how to choose. Several questions can guide you:

- What is your purpose in conducting the study?
- What is the nature of your findings and interpretations?
- Who is/are your audience(s)?
- What are potential uses?
- What voice will be appropriate?
- What trade-offs would an alternative approach require?

And remember that an essential criterion of systematic inquiry is transparency, disclosing research to encourage *professional scrutiny and critique* (Shavelson & Towne, 2002), so you put forward your conceptualization, your method, your analyses and interpretations, and your conclusions to your relevant communities of practice and discourse; these communities decide to accept—or not—the version of reality you represent.

PASSIONS AND CLOSING THE LOOP

In Chapter 1 we referred to the passion needed that "spurs and guides us" (Polanyi, 1966, p. 75) in our study of a specific topic. Deep interest in your topic initiates the journey and sustains you through the twists and turns of conceptualizing and designing. The story of another student's research serves to summarize the first phases of the inquiry journey that lead to a proposal. Passion and potential use triggered Nyongani's (2010) study. Aware that many of the poorest children in her country, Malawi, went to school hungry, she also knew that hungry children cannot be good students—thus, her interest in school feeding programs. Her early exploration into the topic revealed that existing programs were funded by external donors and were not sustainable. In fact, a major donor had recently withdrawn funds, shutting down many of the school feeding programs it had supported. Given their importance for breaking through the cycle of poverty, Nyongani asked, how could feeding programs become sustainable in resource-poor communities in Malawi?

Nyongani turned to the literature, where she learned that "involving community members at the onset of programs greatly increases the chances for such programs to be successful and sustainable" (p. 1). But she also learned that community involvement does not automatically happen to ensure a program's success. She referred to community participation as a "contested concept" (p. 21) and settled on a need to change the mind-set of community members to assume ownership of feeding their children. But what tools would facilitate local planning and change? She studied public health policy; she looked into individual and organizational change theory; she explored systems theory. Finally, she found that social marketing offered tools to illuminate motivators and barriers to behavior change. Following is a graphic representation of her conceptual framework.

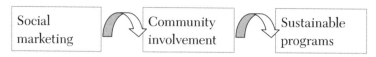

What is noteworthy about Nyongani's (2010) research is that she did not enter it merely to acquire an academic credential; her motivation was her passion to change the way communities in Malawi use resources to ensure that no child goes to school hungry. Nyongani implemented a participatory action research design for her research project, which will implement social marketing tools and explore their effectiveness in building local capacity of communities to feed all their children. As she asserted in her oral defense: "Now 70% of the children in Malawi go to school hungry. We must provide food in schools to ensure that their energy levels are boosted so as to support their cognitive abilities and to promote their regular attendance. The resources are there—we need to use them. By using the tools of social marketing, I can make a change in the social structure of my country."

Nyongani's sincere concern that communities feed all their children will continue to support her as she faces the ups and downs of data collection, analysis, interpretation, and, finally, communicating the results. As we have discussed, seldom do these activities turn out to be easy and straightforward; along with the joys of discovery, she will likely encounter forks and blocks in the road. Probably, as she massages her data, she will revisit the conceptual framework, questioning the connections and definitions she started with. She will learn that the data inform what has become an evolving framework. As during the proposal stages, she will need to rely on her care and passion for the issue to sustain her to her destination.

Often data analysis and interpretation yield discoveries that close the loop by confirming, elaborating, expanding, and modifying the theoretical and conceptual connections you saw at the outset. For example, recall Aysen Kose's (2010) study of how school counselors enact overall school leadership practice for schoolwide improvement. Her lens of distributed leadership proved generative for making sense of her data, but she also saw that this kind of leadership is rare. She learned that to improve their schools, counselors need to be strong advocates for all students, make their practices visible, and build coherence across departments.

In other research studies, your analysis and interpretation of the data yield a very different story, one that asks you to adjust the lens of the conceptual framework. Rallis remembers a student who wanted to understand African American female students who achieved success despite poverty and the challenges of attending a large urban high school. Her conceptual lens was *resilience theory* (see, e.g., Masten, 1994), which suggests strategies, or protective factors, for coping with threatening, stressful, or adverse conditions. She interviewed young women who had graduated from a high school that had been labeled as "troubled" and filled with "at-risk" youth to learn how they coped. To her pleasant surprise, her participants did not see themselves as coping or needing protective factors but, rather, as motivated and accomplished. Her analysis and interpretation of the data took her back to her original framework; she replaced *resilience* with *self-efficacy*

(Bandura, 1977) as a theoretical lens to view the experiences of these young women. In both cases, the researchers closed the loop by reexamining their conceptual frameworks. And in both cases, their passion for their topics carried them to insight and greater understanding.

We have come full circle—you chose your topic, issue, problem, and question for a reason, and your interest in that subject must be strong enough to carry you through the process to information use and knowledge production—knowledge that can, in some way, contribute to improving the human condition. You may note that you cannot control use; you can only seek to promote use through your choices. So, go forth, dear inquirers, with this advice: *Show up, pay attention, tell the truth, and let go of the results.*

Learning Activity 8.1. Connecting with Other Audiences

You've delivered your paper to the professor. Now ask yourself: Who else might be interested? Who else do you want to reach? What groups might have the power to act on what you have learned? The purpose of considering these questions is to generate potential important audiences. Your next step is to design communication formats that will "speak" to these differing audiences. A skit? An instructional manual? A policy brief? A blog post?

FOR FURTHER READING

↪ Kline, R. B. (2008). *Becoming a behavioral science researcher: A guide to producing research that matters*. New York: Guilford Press.

↪ Lindblom, C. (1990). *Inquiry and change*. New Haven, CT: Yale University Press.

↪ Lindblom, C. E., & Cohen, D. K. (Eds.). (1979). *Usable knowledge*. New Haven, CT: Yale University Press.

↪ Patton, M. Q. (2010). *Developmental evaluation: Applying complexity concepts to enhance innovation and use*. New York: Guilford Press.

References

Argyris, C. (1993). *On organizational learning.* Cambridge, MA: Blackwell.

Argyris, C., & Schön, D. A. (1978). *Organizational learning: A theory of action perspective.* San Francisco: Jossey-Bass.

Bandura, A. (1977). Self-efficacy: Toward a unifying theory of behavioral change. *Psychological Review, 84*(2), 191–215.

Bargar, R. R., & Duncan, J. K. (1982). Cultivating creative endeavor in doctoral research. *Journal of Higher Education, 53*(1), 1–31.

Becker, H. S. (1967). Whose side are we on? *Social Problems, 14*(3), 239–247.

Belenky, M. F., Clinchy, B. M., Goldberger, N. R., & Tarule, J. M. (1997). *Women's ways of knowing: The development of self, voice, and mind.* New York: Basic Books.

Berger, P. L., & Luckmann, T. (1967). *The social construction of reality: A treatise in the sociology of knowledge.* New York: Anchor Books, Doubleday.

Bloom, B. S. (Ed.). (1985). *Developing talent in young people.* New York: Ballantine Books.

Blumer, H. (1954). What is wrong with social theory? *American Sociological Review, 19,* 3–10.

Booth, W. C., Colomb, G. G., & Williams, J. M. (2008). *The craft of research* (3rd ed.). Chicago: University of Chicago Press.

Bowen, G. A. (2006). Grounded theory and sensitizing concepts. *International Journal of Qualitative Methods, 5*(3), 2–9.

Bredo, E. (2006). Conceptual confusion and educational psychology. In E. Anderman, P. H. Winne, P. A. Alexander, & L. Corno (Eds.), *Handbook of educational psychology* (2nd ed.). Mahwah, NJ: Erlbaum.

Brunk-Chavez, B. L., & Foster, H. (2010a). *Explorations: A guided inquiry into writing—An overview and TOC.* Retrieved July 6, 2010, from *http://works.bepress.com/beth_brunk_chavez/13.*

Brunk-Chavez, B. L., & Foster, H. (2010b). *Explorations: A guided inquiry into writing—Chapter 1: The nature and process of inquiry.* Retrieved July 6, 2010, from *http://works.bepress.com/beth_brunk_chavez/12.*

Burke, P. J. (2009). *The elements of inquiry: A guide for consumers and producers of research.* Glendale, CA: Pyrczak.

Burrell, G., & Morgan, G. (1979). *Sociological paradigms and organizational analysis.* London: Heinemann.

Carr-Chellman, A. A. (1998). Systemic change: Critically reviewing the literature. *Educational Research and Evaluation, 4*(4), 369–394.

Charmaz, K. (2003). Grounded theory: Objectivist and constructivist methods. In N. K. Denzin & Y. S. Lincoln (Eds.), *Strategies for qualitative inquiry* (2nd ed., pp. 249–291). Thousand Oaks, CA: Sage.

Chilisa, B. (2009). Indigenous African-centered ethics. In D. M. Mertons & P. E. Ginsberg (Eds.), *The handbook of social science research ethics* (pp. 407–425). Thousand Oaks, CA: Sage.

Cooper, H. M. (1988). Organizing knowledge syntheses: A taxonomy of literature reviews. *Knowledge in Society, 1*(1), 104–126.

Council of Graduate Schools in the United States. (1977). *The doctor of philosophy degree: A policy statement.* Washington, DC: Author.

Cousins, J. B., & Whitmore, E. (1998). Framing participatory evaluation. *New Directions for Evaluation, 80,* 5–23.

Davies, D., & Dodd, J. (2002). Qualitative research and the question of rigor. *Qualitative Health Research, 12*(2), 279–289.

Dewey, J. (1896). The reflex arc concept in psychology. *Psychological Review, 3,* 357–370.

Dewey, J. (1938). *Logic: The theory of inquiry.* New York: Holt.

DiMaggio, P. J., & Powell, W. W. (1991). Introduction. In W. W. Powell & P. J. DiMaggio (Eds.), *The new institutionalism in organizational analysis* (pp. 1–38). Chicago: University of Chicago Press.

Elmore, R. (2000). *Building a new structure for school leadership.* Washington, DC: Albert Shanker Institute.

Erickson, E. H. (1959). *Identity and the life cycle.* New York: International Universities Press.

Evered, R., & Louis, M. R. (1981). Alternative perspectives in the organizational sciences. *Academy of Management Review, 6*, 385–391.

Foucault, M. (1977). *Discipline and punish: The birth of the prison* (A. Sheridan, Trans.). New York: Vintage Books.

Freire, P. (1970). *Pedagogy of the oppressed.* New York: Seabury Press.

Gardner, H. (1993). *Frames of mind: The theory of multiple intelligences* (2nd ed.). New York: Basic Books.

Gardner, H. (1999). *Intelligence reframed: Multiple intelligences for the 21st century.* New York: Basic Books.

Gardner, H., & Hatch, T. (1989). Multiple intelligences go to school: Educational implications of the theory of multiple intelligences. *Educational Researcher, 18*(8), 4–9.

Gladwell, M. (2000). *The tipping point: How little things can make a big difference.* New York: Little, Brown.

Gopnik, A., Meltzoff, A. N., & Kuhl, P. K. (2001). *The scientist in the crib: What early learning tells us about the mind.* New York: Perennial.

Guillemin, M., & Gillam, L. (2004). Ethics, reflexivity, and "ethically important moments" in research. *Qualitative Inquiry, 10*(2), 261–280.

Gunzenhauser, M. G., & Gerstl-Pepin, C. (2006). Engaging graduate education: A pedagogy for epistemological and theoretical diversity. *Review of Higher Education, 29*(3), 319–346.

Hemmings, A. (2006). Great ethical divides: Bridging the gap between institutional review boards and researchers. *Educational Researcher, 35*(4), 12–18.

Hostetler, K. (2005). What is "good" education research? *Educational Researcher, 34*(6), 16–21.

Johnston, J. S. (2006). *Inquiry and education: John Dewey and the quest for democracy.* Albany: State University of New York Press.

Kaplan, A. (2005). The conduct of inquiry. In C. C. Lundberg & C. A. Young (Eds.), *Foundations for inquiry: Choices and trade-offs in the organizational sciences* (pp. 144–151). Stanford, CA: Stanford University Press. (Original work published 1964)

Keller, E. F. (1983). *A feeling for the organism: The life and work of Barbara McClintock.* New York: Freeman.

Kidder, T. (1993). *Old friends.* Boston: Houghton Mifflin.

Knight, P. T. (2002). *Small-scale research: Pragmatic inquiry in social science and the caring professions.* London: Sage.

Kolb, A. Y., & Kolb, D. A. (2005). *Kolb Learning Style Inventory version 3.1: Technical specifications.* Boston: Haygroup.

Kolb, D. A. (1984). *Experiential learning: Experience as the source of learning and development*. Englewood Cliffs, NJ: Prentice Hall.

Kose, A. (2010). *Analysis of school counselors' leadership practices through the lens of distributed leadership*. Unpublished doctoral dissertation, University of Massachusetts, Amherst.

Kuhn, T. (1962). *The structure of scientific revolutions*. Chicago: University of Chicago Press.

Kuntz, A. M. (2010). Representing representation. *International Journal of Qualitative Studies in Education, 23*(4), 423–434.

Lave, J., & Wenger, E. (1991). *Situated learning: Legitimate peripheral participation*. Cambridge, UK: Cambridge University Press.

Leshem, S., & Trafford, V. (2007). Overlooking the conceptual framework. *Innovations in Education and Teaching International, 44*(1), 93–105.

Levinson, D. J., with Darrow, C. N., & Klein, E. B. (1978). *Seasons of a man's life*. New York: Random House.

Levinson, D. J., with Levinson, J. D. (1996). *Seasons of a woman's life*. New York: Knopf.

Lewin, K. (1951). *Field theory in social science: Selected theoretical papers* (D. Cartwright, Ed.). New York: Harper & Row.

Lindblom, C. E., & Cohen, D. K. (Eds.). (1979). *Usable knowledge*. New Haven, CT: Yale University Press.

Lundberg, C. C., & Young, C. A. (Eds.). (2005). *Foundations for inquiry: Choices and trade-offs in the organizational sciences*. Stanford, CA: Stanford Business Books.

MacIntyre, A. (1981). *After virtue*. Notre Dame, IN: University of Notre Dame Press.

Mark, M. M., Henry, G. T., & Julnes, G. (2000). *Evaluation: An integrated framework for understanding, guiding, and improving public and nonprofit policies and programs*. San Francisco: Jossey-Bass.

Marshall, C., & Rossman, G. B. (2011). *Designing qualitative research* (5th ed.). Thousand Oaks, CA: Sage.

Martin, I. (2010, November). *The role of program evaluation in supporting and sustaining state-level school counseling programs: A cross-case analysis of best practices*. Paper presented at the annual meeting of the American Evaluation Association, San Antonio, TX.

Maslowe, A. (1970). *Motivation and personality*. New York: Harper & Row.

Masten, A. S. (1994). Resilience in individual development: Successful adaptation despite risk and adversity. In M. Wang & E. Gordon (Eds.), *Risk and resilience in inner city America: Challenges and prospects* (pp. 3–25). Hillsdale, NJ: Erlbaum.

Militello, M., Rallis, S. F., & Goldring, E. B. (2009). *Leading with inquiry and action: How principals improve teaching and learning.* Thousand Oaks, CA: Corwin.

Mishler, E. G. (1990). Validation in inquiry-guided research: The role of exemplars in narrative studies. *Harvard Educational Review, 60*(4), 415–442.

Mishler, E. G. (2000). Validation in inquiry-guided research: The role of exemplars in narrative studies. In B. M. Brizuela, J. P. Stewart, R. G. Carillo, & J. G. Berger (Eds.), *Acts of inquiry in qualitative research* (*Harvard Educational Review*, Reprint Series No. 34, pp. 119–145). Cambridge, MA: Harvard Educational Review.

National Commission for the Protection of Human Subjects of Biomedical and Behavioral Research. (1979). *The Belmont Report: Ethical principles and guidelines for the protection of human subjects of research.* Washington, DC: Department of Health, Education and Welfare.

Nixon, J., & Sikes, P. (2003). Introduction: Reconceptualizing the debate. In P. Sikes, J. Nixon, & W. Carr (Eds.), *The moral foundations of educational research: Knowledge, inquiry and values* (pp. 1–5). Philadelphia: Open University Press.

Noddings, N. (1984). *Caring: A feminine approach to ethics and moral education.* Berkeley: University of California Press.

Noddings, N. (1995). *Philosophy of education.* Boulder, CO: Westview.

Nyongani, M. (2010). *Social marketing school feeding: Sustainability, community involvement, and social marketing.* Unpublished comprehensive examination, University of Massachusetts Amherst.

Nystrand, M. (1982). *What writers know: The language, process, and structure of written discourse.* New York: Academic Press.

Patton, M. Q. (2008). *Utilization-focused evaluation* (4th ed.). Thousand Oaks, CA: Sage.

Peirce, C. S. (1992). *Reasoning and the logic of things: The Cambridge conferences lectures of 1898* (K. L. Ketner, Ed.). Cambridge, MA: Harvard University Press. (Original work published 1898)

Perry, W. G., Jr. (1970). *Forms of intellectual and ethical development in the college years: A scheme.* New York: Holt, Rinehart & Winston.

Phillips, D. C. (2006). A guide for the perplexed: Scientific educational research, methodolatry, and the gold versus platinum standards. *Educational Research Review, 1,* 15–26.

Piaget, J. (1953). *The child's construction of reality.* London: Routledge & Kegan Paul.

Polanyi, M. (1966). *The tacit dimension.* London: Routledge & Kegan Paul.

Preskill, H., & Boyle, S. (2008). A multidisciplinary model of evaluation capacity building. *American Journal of Evaluation, 29,* 443–460.

Punch, M. (1994). Politics and ethics in qualitative research. In N. K. Denzin & Y. S. Lincoln (Eds.), *Handbook of qualitative research* (pp. 83–97). Thousand Oaks, CA: Sage.

Pycha, A. (n.d.). [Review of the book *The scientist in the crib*]. Retrieved April 6, 2009, from *http://brainconnection.posisscience.com/topics/?main=bkrev/gopnik-scientist.*

Rallis, S. F. (2006a, August). *Considering rigor and probity: Qualitative pathways to credible evidence.* Paper presented at What Constitutes Credible Evidence in Evaluation and Applied Research?, Claremont Graduate University Stauffer Symposium, Claremont, CA.

Rallis, S. F. (2006b, October). *A litmus test for scientifically-based research in education: Reasoning with rigor and probity.* Invited plenary at the annual meeting of the Northeastern Educational Research Association, Kerhonkson, NY.

Rallis, S. F. (2010). "That is NOT what's happening at Horizon!": Ethics and misrepresenting knowledge in text. *International Journal of Qualitative Studies in Education, 23*(4), 435–448.

Rallis, S. F., & Goldring, E. B. (2000). *Principals of dynamic schools: Taking charge of change* (2nd ed.). Thousand Oaks, CA: Corwin.

Rallis, S. F., & Rossman, G. B. (2000). Dialogue for learning: Evaluator as a critical friend. In R. K. Hopkins (Ed.), *How and why language matters in evaluation* (New Directions in Program Evaluation, Vol. 86, pp. 81–92). San Francisco: Jossey-Bass.

Rallis, S. F., & Rossman, G. B. (2003, November). *Innovation and emergence in qualitative evaluation.* Invited plenary at the annual meeting of the American Evaluation Association, Reno, NV.

Rallis, S. F., & Rossman, G. B. (2004, April). *Trustworthiness: Beyond procedures to probity.* Paper presented at the annual meeting of the American Educational Research Association, San Diego, CA.

Rallis, S. F., & Rossman, G. B. (2010). Caring reflexivity. *International Journal of Qualitative Studies in Education, 23*(4), 495–499.

Rallis, S. F., Rossman, G. B., Cobb, C. D., Reagan, T. G., & Kuntz, A. M. (2008). *Leading dynamic schools: How to create and implement ethical policies.* Thousand Oaks, CA: Corwin.

Rallis, S. F., Rossman, G. B., & Gajda, R. (2007). Trustworthiness in evaluation practice: An emphasis on the relational. *Evaluation and Program Planning, 30,* 401–409.

Rawls, J. (1971). *A theory of justice.* Cambridge, MA: Harvard University Press.

Regaignon, D. R. (2009). Traction: Transferring analysis across the curriculum. *Pedagogy: Critical Approaches to Teaching Literature, Language, Composition, and Culture, 9*(1), 121–133.

Rein, M. (1970). *Social policy: Issues of choice and change.* New York: Random House.

Rosenthal, R. (1994). Science and ethics in conducting, analyzing, and reporting psychological research. *Psychological Research, 5*(3), 127–134.

Rossman, G. B., & Evans, D. R. (2002). *Using the work and words of other authors: A guide to APA style for international students—and others.* Amherst, MA: Center for International Education. Retrieved November 22, 2010, from *www.umass.edu/cie/Themes/#themepage.*

Rossman, G. B., & Rallis, S. F. (1998). *Learning in the field: An introduction to qualitative research.* Thousand Oaks, CA: Sage.

Rossman, G. B., & Rallis, S. F. (2003). *Learning in the field: An introduction to qualitative research* (2nd ed.). Thousand Oaks, CA: Sage.

Rossman, G. B., & Rallis, S. F. (2010). Everyday ethics: Reflections on practice. *International Journal of Qualitative Studies in Education, 23*(4), 379–391.

Rossman, G. B., Rallis, S. F. (2012). *Learning in the field: An introduction to qualitative research* (3rd ed.). Thousand Oaks, CA: Sage.

Rossman, G. B., Rallis, S. F., & Kuntz, A. M. (2010). Validity: Mapping diverse perspectives. In E. Baker, B. McGaw, & P. Peterson (Eds.), *The international encyclopedia of education* (3rd ed., pp. 505–513). Amsterdam: Elsevier.

Scheffler, I. (1965). *Conditions of knowledge: An introduction to epistemology and education.* Chicago: University of Chicago Press.

Schön, D. A. (1983). *The reflective practitioner: How professionals think in action.* New York: Basic Books.

Schram, T. H. (2006). *Conceptualizing and proposing qualitative research* (2nd ed.). Upper Saddle River, NJ: Pearson Merrill Prentice Hall.

Schratz, M., & Walker, R. (1995). *Research as social change: New opportunities for qualitative research.* London: Routledge.

Seiber, J. (2004). Informed consent. In M. S. Lewis-Beck, A. Bryman, & T. F. Liao (Eds.), *The Sage encyclopedia of social science research methods* (Vol. 1, pp. 493–497). Thousand Oaks, CA: Sage.

Senge, P. M. (1994). *The fifth discipline: The art and practice of the learning organization* (2nd ed.). New York: Currency Doubleday.

Shavelson, R., & Towne, L. (Eds.). (2002). *Scientific research in education.* Washington, DC: Committee on Scientific Principles for Education Research, National Research Council.

Sikes, P., & Goodson, I. (2003). Living research: Thoughts on educational research as moral practice. In P. Sikes, J. Nixon, & W. Carr (Eds.), *The moral foundations of educational research: Knowledge, inquiry and values* (pp. 32–51). Berkshire, UK: Open University Press.

Slife, B. D., & Williams, R. N. (1995). *What's behind the research?: Discovering hidden assumptions in the behavioral sciences.* Thousand Oaks, CA: Sage.

Spillane, J. P. (2004). *Distributed leadership: What's all the hoopla?* Chicago: Northwestern University, Institute for Policy Research.

Spillane, J. P., & Miele, D. B. (2007). Evidence in practice: A framing of the terrain. In P. A. Moss (Ed.), *Evidence and decision making: The 106th yearbook of the National Society for the Study of Education* (Part I, pp. 46–73). Malden, MA: Blackwell.

Strike, K., Haller, E., & Soltis, J. (1998). *The ethics of school administration* (2nd ed.). New York: Teachers College Press.

Van Maanen, J. (1983). The moral fix: On the ethics of fieldwork. In R. Emerson (Ed.), *Contemporary field research: A collection of readings* (pp. 363–376). Prospect Heights, IL: Waveland.

Vygotsky, L. S. (1978). *Mind in society: The development of higher psychological processes.* Cambridge, MA: Harvard University Press.

Warnock, J. (2008, November/December). [Review of the book *Leading dynamic schools: How to create and implement ethical policies*]. Retrieved November 1, 2010, from *www.naesp.org/resources/2/Principal/2008/N-Dp50.pdf.*

Watson, J. D. (1968). *The double helix: A personal account of the discovery of the structure of DNA.* New York: Atheneum.

Weick, K. (1979). *The social psychology of organizing* (2nd ed.). Reading, MA: Addison-Wesley.

Weick, K. (1995). *Sensemaking in organizations.* Newbury Park, CA: Sage.

Weiss, C. H. (1998). *Evaluation: Methods for studying programs and policies* (2nd ed.). Upper Saddle River, NJ: Prentice Hall.

Williams, M. (2001). *Problems of knowledge: A critical introduction to epistemology.* Oxford, UK: Oxford University Press.

Wolf, M. (1992). *A thrice told tale: Feminism, postmodernism, and ethnographic responsibility.* Stanford, CA: Stanford University Press.

Author Index

179

Subject Index

Page numbers followed by *f* indicate figure, *t* indicate table

About the Authors

Sharon F. Rallis, EdD, is Dwight W. Allen Distinguished Professor of Education Policy and Reform at the University of Massachusetts Amherst, where she is also Director of the Center for Education Policy. Dr. Rallis has coauthored 10 books, including *Learning in the Field: An Introduction to Qualitative Research* (with Gretchen B. Rossman; now in its third edition) and several on leadership—*Principals of Dynamic Schools: Taking Charge of Change* (with Ellen B. Goldring), *Dynamic Teachers: Leaders of Change* (with Gretchen B. Rossman), *Leading Dynamic Schools: How to Create and Implement Ethical Policies* (with Gretchen B. Rossman and others), and *Leading with Inquiry and Action: How Principals Improve Teaching and Learning* (with Matthew Militello and Ellen B. Goldring). Her numerous articles, book chapters, edited volumes, and technical reports address issues of research and evaluation methodology, ethical practice in research and evaluation, education policy and leadership, and school reform. A past president of the American Evaluation Association, Dr. Rallis has been involved with education and evaluation for over three decades as a teacher, counselor, principal, researcher, program evaluator, director of a major federal school reform initiative, and an elected school board member. Currently, her teaching includes courses on inquiry, program evaluation, qualitative methodology, and organizational theory. Her research has focused on the local implementation of programs driven by federal, state, or district policies. As external evaluator or principal investigator (PI), she has studied a variety of domestic and international policy and reform efforts, such as alternative professional development for leaders, collaborations between agencies responsible for educating incarcerated or institutionalized youth, initiatives supporting inclusive education for children and youth with disabilities, local school governance and leadership, and labor–management relations in school districts. Dr. Rallis's work with students on evaluation and qualitative methodology has taken her as far as Afghanistan and Palestine.

Gretchen B. Rossman, PhD, is Chair of the Department of Educational Policy, Research and Administration and Professor of International Education at the Center for International Education at the University of Massachusetts Amherst. With an international reputation as a qualitative methodologist, Dr. Rossman has expertise in qualitative research design and methods, mixed methods monitoring and evaluation, and inquiry in education. She has coauthored nine books, two of which are editions of major qualitative research texts—*Learning in the Field* (with Sharon F. Rallis; see above) and *Designing Qualitative Research* (with Catherine Marshall; fifth edition)—both widely used guides to qualitative inquiry. Her numerous articles, book chapters, and technical reports focus on methodological issues in qualitative research syntheses, validity in qualitative research, mixed methods evaluation practice, and ethical research practice, as well as the analysis and evaluation of educational reform initiatives both in the United States and internationally. Dr. Rossman has served as PI or co-PI on several international projects in countries such as Azerbaijan, India, Malawi, Palestine, Senegal, Tanzania, and The Gambia, as well as external evaluator on several domestic projects, including a U.S. Department of Education–funded reform initiative, a National Science Foundation–funded middle-grades science initiative, and a number of projects implementing more inclusive practices for students with disabilities. She regularly presents papers at the annual meetings of the American Evaluation Association, the American Educational Research Association (AERA), and the Comparative and International Education Society, and served a 2-year term as program co-chair (with Sharon F. Rallis) for the qualitative research section of AERA's Division on Research Methodology.

Drs. Rallis and Rossman have had a productive collaborative career as coauthors, co-instructors, and mentors of graduate students. They have written together on ethical research practice, ethical policy implementation, mixed methods evaluation practice, validity in qualitative inquiry, and other methodological issues. They currently teach a course together at the University of Massachusetts Amherst— *Introduction to Inquiry*—that is required for all incoming doctoral students and forms the basis for this book. Mentoring graduate students informs their writing, and they regularly invite graduate students to write with them. They have worked together with graduate students from Afghanistan, Azerbaijan, Bhutan, China, India, Kenya, Kyrgyzstan, Malawi, Pakistan, Palestine, Sierra Leone, Tajikistan, Thailand, Uzbekistan, and the United States. This work has taken them on journeys ("road trips") around the globe, where they have facilitated workshops and made presentations to practitioners and academic audiences.